Cancer Is a Bitch

Cancer Is a Bitch

(Or, I'd Rather Be
Having a Midlife Crisis)

GAIL KONOP BAKER

Da Capo
LIFE
LONG

A Member of the Perseus Books Group

Designed by Pauline Brown
Set in 11.5 point Minion by the Perseus Books Group

Library of Congress Cataloging-in-Publication Data

Baker, Gail Konop.
Cancer is a bitch : or I'd rather be having a midlife crisis /
Gail Konop Baker. — 1st ed.
p. cm.
ISBN 978-0-7382-1162-6 (alk. paper)
1. Baker, Gail Konop—Health.
2. Breast—Cancer—Patients—Wisconsin—Biography. I. Title.
RC280.B8B347 2008
362.196'994490092—dc22
[B]
2008015161

First Da Capo Press edition 2008

Published by Da Capo Press
A Member of the Perseus Books Group
www.dacapopress.com

Da Capo Press books are available at special discounts for bulk purchases in the U.S. by corporations, institutions, and other organizations. For more information, please contact the Special Markets Department at the Perseus Books Group, 2300 Chestnut Street, Suite 200, Philadelphia, PA, 19103, or call (800) 810-4145, ext. 5000, or e-mail special.markets@perseusbooks.com.

10 9 8 7 6 5 4 3 2 1

For Rick, Ali, Abby, and Andrew with
adoration and affection

In loving memory of Ann Kelley
and Richard Konop

Author's Note

To all the women, men, and children who have been pierced by cancer's insidious claw and to those whose diagnoses were and are more severe than mine and to all the people who do not have adequate access to health care and/or the time and resources to recover from their illnesses, my heart goes out to you and your loved ones. I wrote this book with all of you in mind. And, in a small effort to honor you, a portion of the proceeds from *Cancer Is a Bitch* will be donated to the National Breast Cancer Coalition and the Wisconsin Well Woman Program.

[*one*]

More
Important
Things to Do

I'M PICTURING CARRIE on *Sex and the City* cross-legged on her bed in sexy boy-cut undies and a cleavage revealing push-up bra, her hair professionally disheveled, seductively sucking on a melting Popsicle. She made writing look like a must-have accessory, the quirky detail that set her apart from other women. All the years I watched that show, I thought, I could do that. I should have done that. I lived in New York City. I had sex. I had girlfriends who called me frantic in the middle of the night complaining about their Mr. Bigs not being so big. I could write witty sentences verging

on the annoying. I could work a Popsicle with the best
of them. But as much as I see Carrie out of the corner of
my eye as I type, I'm not Carrie. Not by a long shot. I'm
married. I'm the mother of three. I live in Wisconsin. I
don't own boy-cut undies and instead of baring my relationship with men and shoes, I'm baring my relationship with breast cancer.

I'll start in the middle: Winter 2006:

I'm sitting topless in the oncologist's office on Valentine's Day. Cancer is a bitch. It doesn't give a shit about
holidays. Doesn't give a shit when the oncologist gently
presses his thick hairy fingers near the wound above
my nipple, tears burn the raw edges of my puffy eyes,
dribble down my cheeks, and roll past blood-caked
stitches, landing in a puddle in the space between the
oncologist's cold wedding band and my warm flesh.
"Still swollen," he says and I hate him. Hate that I'm
swollen, hate that I'm here on Valentine's Day instead
of at Victoria's Secret buying the cleavage-enhancing
Miracle Bra that *Redbook* recommended for guaranteed flawless shape. Think if I'd followed their "Sizzle
for Your Sweetie" advice, I would be slipping into a red
dress, on my way to a romantic dinner, wouldn't be
hearing the oncologist saying, "Even though the surgeon got clean margins, your risk of invasive cancer is
four to five times greater than the average woman."
Wouldn't be afraid to look at my flawed breast under
the harsh fluorescent light.

It all began the morning of my annual mammogram a few weeks earlier in January. Over breakfast my nine-year-old son Alex and I discussed the puppy he'd been begging for, ever since the death of our dog that past Thanksgiving. Now that I'd finished my novel (about a woman who finds a lump in her breast and wonders if she's lived a meaningful life), I was ready to consider a new pet at the close of what had been a stressful, busy year—the dog dying, my husband, Mike's, slow-healing knee surgery, and our oldest daughter, Anna's, college application process. A nearly straight-A student with SAT scores comparable to my Ivy League radiologist husband's, a singer, a dancer, and a cross-country runner, and she'd been rejected early-decision by Dartmouth, his alma matter. Dartmouth had been a source of tension for us all the way back to when Mike brought me home to his mother, who was disappointed that I wasn't the blond-bobbed, Episcopalian Dartmouth grad she'd sent him to college to meet. Instead, I was a wavy-haired, curvy, Jewish, wanna-be poet who lived in the East Village and had gone to an "experimental" college (even I wondered what she could possibly make of me).

So when Anna said she didn't want to apply to Dartmouth, I said if she didn't want to, she shouldn't; and Mike said I was undermining him, turning her against *his* school and that I obviously didn't understand the whole "Ivy League thing." Our middle daughter, Maddy—also in high school and panicked by her sister's panic—signed up for more clubs, SAT prep, and dance team, while Alex was playing indoor soccer and basketball, both at opposite ends of town. As if that wasn't enough, all year I'd felt pressure from my agent to send her my new manuscript.

But that morning, I dropped Alex off at school, brought the newspaper with me to my mammogram, and as I waited in the cubicle for the technician to tell me to get dressed and go home, I circled "healthy, lovable, mixed-breed pups free to good home," and thought about how much more time I would have now that the other college applications were in the mail and my new novel was complete. I'd start back at yoga and cook more elaborate dinners and do something about the war in Iraq and global warming and match all the un-matched socks instead of stuffing them into that old bureau at the top of the stairs—when the technician peeked in and said, "We need to get a few more films."

"Not to worry," she said, as she whisked me down the hall smiling, continuing the story about her grand-son or granddaughter or grandsomething doing some-thing grand. "Doctors' wives make everybody nervous," she said and rolled her eyes, gesturing for me to slip my arm out of my gown.

After seven films and more cubicle waiting, I folded up the want ads, picked up a magazine featuring a young woman with inoperable lung cancer, put down the magazine, stood and counted to a hundred forward and backward. I'd had a couple of breast scares before, a core biopsy and a wide excision, both indicating cellular changes, but ultimately benign. I worried about my breasts, but still, I felt impatient with all this wasted time when I had more important things to do.

The technician poked her head back into the stall. "Dr. Evans wants to talk to you," she said. No small talk, no smile as she led me into the viewing room.

I stood next to Henry, one of my husband's radiologist partners and a friend of ours for years. I knew his wife, his children; we'd shared numerous occasions— weddings, graduations, anniversaries, funerals. As he pointed to an illuminated x-ray of my breast, all swirly white clouds and dissipating smoke plumes, a thin red arrow marking a teeny tiny cluster of white specks, he said, "See, that's what I'm concerned about. Those calcifications are new and just to be safe I think we should biopsy. . . . "

He choked and winced, looking so pained to have to tell *me* this news that I said, "This must be awkward for you."

He nodded and said, "Okay?"

And I wondered, Was he asking me my opinion? Was there a choice? Was this a trick question? Was there an answer that would make this go away?

He swallowed so loudly, I felt it in *my* throat.

"Okay," I said, wanting to make *him* feel better.

Murmuring *okay okay okay okay* all the way down the hall, in the elevator, into the parking lot, where I stood, lost, unable to find my car, the ink from the crumpled newspaper bleeding into my hand.

two

Does Biopsy
Mean No Puppy?

CHEST DOWN ON a padded table, head cocked sideways, right breast hanging through a peekaboo hole, one arm hooked around my matted hair, the other arm twisted pinky side out along my side, the nurse positions me from below as the clear-plastic compression paddles squish my flesh into place.

"Are you comfortable?" she asks and swabs my breast with betadine.

I'm not sure how to answer that. I'm strapped to a surgical bed by my boob. I'm expected to be still while a long thick needle excavates questionable cells. I'm contorted. I'm scared. But none of that is her fault so I nod, the stiff sheet scratching my cheek, a little bit of drool trickling into my ear.

"First, I'm going to numb you," she says and cocks the needle into the antiseptic air, dribbling a bubble of fluid out the tip, and pierces my skin.

"Numb is good," I tell both of us.

She scootches up a chair near my head and says, "Aren't you a writer?"

I nod as Pete, another of my husband's radiology partners, approaches the table. "Are you ready?"

He isn't a close friend like Henry, who'd read my mammogram. But when I first moved to Madison, I was in a book group with his wife. One time we read a "literary erotic" novel called *Eat Me,* and we all drank too much wine and shared too much, something involving sushi and fishnets and marzipan—was that something from the book or his wife?

"Ready," I say. The worn pale-blue patient gown barely veils my rigid body, and I remember that the last time I saw Pete was at the annual holiday party and I was dancing to "Love Shack" in a tight black dress and stilettos.

"What's your book about?" the nurse asks, patting my arm as if I'm three, and I'm grateful and worried that I've engendered such tenderness.

"A woman who finds a lump in her breast," I say above the whir of the machine. I feel pressure but no pain, trying not to think about the needle, trying to picture my children romping on a beach, a peaceful image I've used in yoga class to pull me out of my ruminating head. I see the tide rolling in and in and in and think, Shiva, the Hindu God of regeneration, a mantra that means one thing must die for another to be born. . . .

•   •   •

"Does this make my boobs look too big?" my fifteen-year-old middle daughter Maddy had asked, three shirts and two bras into her evening fashion show the night before. I was lying on her bed, thinking about how distorted the ceiling looked through her satin canopy, all translucent cracks and amorphous shards.

"Try the green shirt with the *other* bra," I answered.

Maddy and I often had these boob conversations because although she was blond and blue-eyed like Mike, she was built like me, small but busty, and she knew that I knew how hard it was to find the right clothes—too fitted and you looked like a sexpot, too baggy and you looked matronly. We had hard figures to dress, hard figures to rationalize.

"I can hear you," my older, less busty daughter Anna shouted from her room.

"Your breasts look great in everything," I said to Maddy, the word "breasts" clinging to the back of my throat. The only time I'd felt entirely comfortable with my breasts was when I was nursing. Otherwise, I'd always had a love/hate relationship with them. The first time Jake Jabowitz felt me up in eighth grade, I thought I loved him, until I found out he told all the other boys I had great tits. But on my daughters, I saw them differently. Perfect sculptures, round and soft and firm and healthy. My stomach flipped.

"That is such a bitch thing for you to say," Anna said to me as she stormed into the room, her large green eyes piercing mine.

I gasped into my fist. Willing myself not to say anything I would regret. Mike and I had decided we'd tell the girls about the procedure later that night, together, and downplay it, and not tell Alex at all. No need to burden them.

"Do you have any idea what a pain in the ass these things are?" Maddy said. "Mom knows."

My face grew too hot as I told myself, Be mature and restrained. "That wasn't meant as a slight to you," I sat up and said as slowly as possible to Anna. "You look great in everything, too. You both do. You're young and beautiful, you have your whole lives in front of you for chrissakes, what the hell are you complaining about? And don't swear at me," I screamed, tears blurring everything.

"What? What's wrong with you?" Anna said.

"Nothing. Nothing. Noth. . . . " My throat catching

in the middle of the third "nothing." "I'm having a b . . . b . . . b . . ." I said, the consonant stuck on my lips.

"A baby?" Anna said.

"A biopsy." The word coming out too loud, too aggressively, making it sound more ominous than I wanted it to.

"*Another* one?" Maddy said.

"What does biopsy mean?" Alex poked his wide-eyed, freckled face in from the hallway.

Shit, why did he have to hear that? "It means. . . ." I hadn't meant to have this conversation. How had this happened? And what *did* it mean? "It means. . . ." He'd go to a friend's house after school tomorrow and I'd watch *Oprah* to recover; and we'd order in pizza for dinner and if all went well, that would be it, everything back to normal. And if not, my defective breast might be the most memorable legacy I would leave my children.

"Does it mean no puppy?" he asked, so gently, he must have known I needed help articulating and I wondered, What kind of mother would allow this, any of this, to happen?

•   •   •

Another whir of the machine reminds me of the table, of me on the table, of life cycles spinning in opposite directions simultaneously. My children's coming-of-age, my aging. I glance at the needle penetrating my yellowed boob and hope biopsy doesn't mean I'll be a burden before they have blossomed.

"Clamp," the nurse warns as Pete shoots a metal staple into my breast.

I shudder at the noise, the clutch of internal force, the fact that I know it's marked so the surgeon can find the spot if it's cancerous. "That's two," I say. "I hope I don't set off any metal detectors."

"You're a good sport," Pete says as he unleashes my body from the paddles.

No, I'm not. Not a good sport, not mature enough to handle this. I want out before the stakes get any higher. I want to turn back the clock. I want to reread *Eat Me*. I want to dance to "Love Shack" in a too-tight dress. I want to call Jake Jabowitz and ask him if he still thinks I have great tits.

"So, what happens to the woman in the novel?" the nurse interrupts my thoughts, wrapping my chest in loose layers of sterile gauze.

"She's, she's, she's. . . . " I want to say "fine," but I'd left her fate ambiguous, thinking that was the more interesting choice. And now I wonder why I hadn't worked that out, because *I* want to know what happens to the woman, as I tie my frayed blue gown around me, slide off the biopsy table, my paper slippers landing on the cold linoleum with a jarring thud.

[*three*]

I'm "It"

I WAS WATCHING *Oprah,* waiting for the results from my core biopsy and of the final From Frumpy to Fabulous unveiling of the housewife from Kalamazoo after the commercial break, when Cancer barged into my family room saying *Sorry sorry sorry sorry, you have ductal carcinoma in situ.*

"Are you sure are you sure are you sure are you sure?" I blabbered, as if that string of words said emphatically enough would overpower the other words. But words were not words. Words were fish and the air a murky cesspool spewing lies. Damn lies!

Like sorry? Cancer didn't mean sorry. It meant, fuck you and your comfort, your complacency, your petty concerns, your smug belief that you deserved to be lucky, to live unscathed. Fuck you and your naïve delusion that you had any, *any* control over the fate of your body.

"It's intermediate grade and we don't know how much is in there," Mike, now home, said in a voice too high, too loud, too soft, too strained, too stricken, too *I'm going to be really nice to you now because I'm afraid you're going to die.*

How could I yearn for his impatient tone?

"The sooner we get *it* out the better," he said, rubbing his hands on his pants so vigorously I thought he thought I thought he could rub *it* away.

I shook my head. "Alex has a basketball tournament and Maddy starts driver's ed tomorrow and Anna has a term paper due and, and . . . we're out of milk . . . and, and, and. . . . " I pointed to the TV, a commercial for Botox, the words IT'S *YOUR* TURN NOW illuminating the screen. ". . . And *Oprah* is over and now I've missed the housewife from Kalamazoo," I said and burst into tears.

But Cancer didn't hear me, didn't see me cry. It was busy moving in, crushing my sternum, throttling my throat, sucker punching my gut, bullying me into submission.

How had I not appreciated my health all those years I didn't have a diagnosis following me everywhere like an annoying sibling, mimicking my every move, mirroring the parts of me that make me feel awkward, ashamed? My diagnosis, a brat, demanding center stage, forcing me to fill my calendar with appointments where I'm weighed and blood pressured and poked and probed, felt up and down and warned about my risk.

I want to be brave. I want to be big. I want to be gracious and cool. I want to be the Audrey Hepburn of cancer. I want to be like that girl who went to my high school, Heather Arnold. Tall and lithe and wide-eyed, she had leukemia and when her long diaphanous white-blond hair fell out, she tied the most gorgeous silk scarves around her delicate head, sloped bell-bottom pants off her jutting hips, wrapped her bony wrists in loose sheaves of silver bangles. She wore it well. She made cancer look sexy. As if the very fact that she wouldn't be here forever made her mysterious and irresistible, more valuable than the rest of us.

But I'm not like Heather. For one thing, I'm not tall. Or bony. And cancer doesn't feel sexy on me. It feels ugly, cankerous, mean, and old. It reminds me that I'll never be twenty again, that time has moved faster and less kindly than I expected. And I'm not wearing it well. I can't figure out how to hold my face anymore, what to do with these weary eyes afraid to stare back at me, this mouth that doesn't know how to smile anymore when smiling feels so foreign, so strange. Why do, how do people, how did I ever smile? when all I can think is *cancer cancer cancer cancer.*

As I sit on the examining table in the internist's office for my pre-op physical a day or two later, I think about Joan Didion's *The Year of Magical Thinking,* how it was praised for its lack of self-pity as I silently chant *poor me poor me poor me.* It takes all of my energy to contain my tears. But I don't know my internist very well, have seen her twice in five years (my two other breast scares that turned out benign). Otherwise, I am almost never sick. No colds, no flus, no aches or pains. I run with my daughters, shoot hoops with my son, practice yoga, eat organic food. I am an armchair nutritionist, a person others consult for health and anti-aging tips, a lifelong subscriber to *Prevention.* I feel that "me" slipping away as I wonder how I could suffer a condition more serious than my chain-smoking nitrate-loving fruit-phobic nonexercising mother-in-law ever experienced. Fuck you, Joan Didion. It wasn't *you* who keeled over before dinner. *Why me why me why me?*

"I looked around my son's kindergarten classroom of twenty-four," the internist says, slicing into my less than stoic thoughts, pressing the cool stethoscope on my back, motioning for me to take a deep breath. "And I thought three of these mothers. . . . " Her sentence trails. She looks at me as if I'm supposed to finish her thought.

"Three?" I say.

"One in eight." She shakes her head and works her finger up my neck to feel for lymph nodes. "Any of *your* friends?"

"No," I say. As she runs her fingers up and down my throat, oddly, I think about when I studied Emerson in graduate school—"I have enjoyed a perfect exhilaration. I am glad to the brink of fear"—and that it reminded me of how I felt when I was a child and played duck, duck, goose and was tagged.

Before I dress, she presses a prescription for Valium into my hand, her eyes more apprehensive than I want them to be. I want her to take it all back, say it isn't true, say: We were wrong, you are fine, no need for surgery, go home, eat a lot of red dye #2, and fritter away the rest of your ridiculously long life. Instead she says, "Don't worry," patting my wrist, tripping over the second syllable in "worry." Making me worried that she can't even say the word and I feel her pity metamorphosize me. I'm "It." I'm goose. I'm giddy. I'm trapped. I'm trembling.

After Mike and I fill my prescription, the whole way home I hum the Rolling Stones song about the mother running for the shelter of her mother's little helper, rattling the pill bottle against my thigh like a tambourine.

[*four*]

Nothing
Has Changed

IN THE HANDFUL of days between pre-op and surgery,
I wake in the cold raw February dawn, stand naked
before the full-length mirror, memorizing the contours
I spent decades criticizing. I shower, shampoo, condition, blow-dry my hair section by section, button myself into a suit I bought in '87 for a job I forgot to
pursue, put on heels and more makeup than I know
how to apply, and tiptoe downstairs to make a nice big
breakfast before anyone awakens because nothing has
changed. I'm the mother. I'm dressed. I'm coiffed. I'm
cooking. I remove a dozen eggs from the refrigerator,

open the carton, study the smooth brown mounds tucked into cardboard nests, and can't remember what to do with eggs.

By the time the children come down, the air is gauzy with the news we shared with them the night before and the singed fumes from the entire loaf of bread I've toasted piece by piece, each one more burnt than the next, and I'm frantically hiding the crispy edges with sloppy globs of mixed-berry jam.

"A suit?" Maddy says.

"Why do you look like that?" Anna asks, eyeing me up and down, her gaze landing on my hair.

I am about to share my hour-long hair-drying method when, out of the corner of my eye, I see jam clinging to my frazzled ends.

"This toast is sick," Alex says, spitting out a mouthful into his hand. "This isn't *your* toast, Mom."

"Be nice to your mother," Mike says, as he enters the kitchen, his bottom lip quivering every time he looks at me.

"No, no, no!" I say. "Do *not* be nice to your mother. I will not tolerate—niceness—now!" My hand slamming into the carton of eggs, flipping them off the counter, the cracked shells and mucoussy innards pooling at my feet.

While the children are at school, I send my novel about the woman who finds a lump in her breast to my agent, telling myself, At least I have my finished novel. I don't mention my health scare to her because she is twenty-five and I worry this news will make her think I'm too old, too risky to handle. I Google *Breast Cancer* obsessively, ductal carcinoma in situ, grades and staging, recurrence rates, hormone therapy. I learn that although DCIS is noninvasive it is often found next to invasive sites, that it can be a precursor to invasive cancer. In a breast cancer chat room, I find a woman who was a six-year noninvasive "survivor," announcing bone metastases. I learn that some women with the combination of my history of biopsies and this diagnosis choose prophylactic mastectomy because it's too stressful to live with the constant threat. I log on to mastectomy sites where breasts are displayed row after row, headless and bottomless, removed and rebuilt like used headlights from an auto body repair shop. I glance down at my still full chest puckering my suit lapels and think, If they have to go, I'll go smaller and perkier, more like Anna, and give my good bras to Maddy, and burn the rest (I always wanted to go braless). I'm feeling more hopeful. Until I Google *Carcinogens* and find toxins everywhere: pesticides in produce; PCPs in fish; hormones in meat and dairy; chlorine in water; automobile and industrial emissions in the air; TVs, cell phones, computers all spewing electromagnetic waves.

I try to picture what to eat, how to breathe, where to go, my eyes landing on the wires and cables tangling into our power-surge protector like snakes. I lift my fingers from the keyboard and think, Leave this venom-pit-posing-as-a-family-room (ha!), pick up the children from school, and take all of us to a safe place where the air is clean, the water purified, and the electromagnetic field outlawed. Step away from the computer, I think, but my pinky inches onto the keyboard, clicks *Toxins in Cosmetics* just a little, lightly, almost doesn't, but it does, and up pops: *Skin is the largest organ and any substance applied to it enters the body unfiltered.* According to a 2004 study published in the Canadian *Journal of Applied Toxicology*, parabens were found in twenty human breast tumors. The products I bought and applied religiously to keep me youthful? My age-defying lotions, overnight miracle creams, hair-like-silk shampoos and conditioners? All likely riddled with parabens: methylparabens, polyparabens, ethylparabens. I think about the parabens penetrating my hair shafts and I run upstairs, strip off my suit, lean over the side of the tub, turn on the water full blast, the faux-herbal blast of hair products stinging my nostrils, mutating more cells for all I know, right this very second . . . when Martha, one of my best friends, taps me on the shoulder, startling me.

"I let myself in," she says, looking all sporty and fit. "You wanna run a half-marathon in New York City this summer?"

I'm thrown by her question. I've told her about the surgery but not how the concept of future baffles me. New York? Summer? Run? What do *those* words have to do with *this* me? "I'm thinking of getting rid of the time bombs," I say and cup my breasts as I flip my sopping head up, foundation running off my face and staining the fluffy white rug.

She doesn't say anything and I think of all the things I admire about her: She rides an old motorcycle to the grocery store; ski jumps with her daughters; changes her own oil; is a triathlete and marathoner and pushes me to run harder and longer and faster than I ever imagine I am capable of. She's way cooler and more daring than I am, and up until this moment I didn't think it mattered that much, but now I worry she won't like this damaged me. And, honestly, I don't blame her.

"Then we'll throw a Goodbye Breasts party," she says, wiping a clump of mascara from my cheek. "And if you lose your hair, I'm shaving my head in solidarity," she says and hugs me, and I'm ashamed and relieved that I underestimated the depth of our friendship.

I troll the streets, looking into the eyes of old people who don't look particularly healthy, who don't look as if they've worried about TOXINS and wonder what they did differently than me. Were they better people? Did they pray? I pray. I picture Mrs. Campbell, my old neighbor who died at ninety-nine, her warm, pie-shaped face, her sturdy gait, the way her face lit up at the crocuses, the strength of her grip on my forearm, her lovely worn accordion neck. I try her sweet expression on my face. I pray to *be* Mrs. Campbell. I pray to live long enough to see my children grown, to see my grandchildren, my great grandchildren, my great great great grandchildren, to be free of my rabid, insatiable desire for more.

I ride the stationary bike in our basement and think, I am Lance Armstrong, I am strong, I am a fighter. When "I Will Survive" comes on the radio, I belt out the chorus and burst into hysterical tears. Why do *I* have to fight? Why can't I just be? And sob like a baby.

When Alex is in bed and the girls are in their rooms, I ask Mike, "Can you get an electromagnetic field detector because between the wireless and the bigger TV, I'm thinking the family room is. . . . "

"Have you been Googling again?"

"We should move to Utah and live off the land. That way we'll know the source of everything we put in our mouths."

"You're going to get up and milk cows at the crack of dawn?"

"No cows. I'm off dairy. I'm thinking all-organic vegetable gardens. . . . "

"Do you remember what happened to the impatiens?" he says, reminding me how I forgot to water them in the heat wave and they died.

"That's *not* the right answer," I say.

We both wait for him to figure out what is. . . .

"What do you want me to say?" His voice so shaky I shudder at the thought of leaving him to grieve without me.

"That I'm going to be okay?" I say, offering him words to try on like the ill-fitting suit I left puddled in the bathroom.

"You're going to be okay," he says, lip quivering.

"Do you really think so?"

"I don't know," he says, his doubt dangling precariously in the taut, uncharted air between us.

"What do you mean, you don't know?" I ask, knowing there is nothing he can say that will make me feel better, that I'm creating an impossible bind by asking him and hating myself but unable to prevent myself from torturing both of us.

I dream of the abyss, of me in the abyss, wake at 2 A.M. in a cold sweat, call my other best friend, Rachel, my wisest friend, the one who maintains the most direct line to God, and ask her, "Is it dark? 'Cause I picture it dark." I choke. I've always been afraid of the dark. She gulps and sighs, says she'll ask the rabbi and get back to me. I try to surrender to sleep, am afraid to sleep, think that sleep is a kind of letting go and letting go is a kind of death and death is dark. I fixate on the one point of light from the neighbors' laundry room and when that goes out, I stumble downstairs, log on to e-mail, and find my agent's reply: *The problem I'm having with the novel is I just don't really care whether the protagonist has breast cancer or not.* There's more, but all I can see is that one line as I stare at the screen, trying not to feel the words stab me, drag myself back upstairs, crawl under the comforter, press my damp face into Mike's back, longing to absorb the measure of his breath and make it my own. I wake up muttering, "I don't know what to do. I don't know what to do," roll out of bed, peel my rumpled suit off the floor, pull it on, and start all over again.

And with every ounce of good mothering common sense I can muster, I scrub nonexistent gook off the kitchen sink with S.O.S pads until my arm cramps, my knuckles bleed, and my warped reflection glares back at me, because I'm the mother. I'm doing what needs to be done! *Nothing* has changed, and when Alex says he'd like a bowling party for his birthday in April, I smile and nod, smile and nod, smileandnodsmileandnod **smileandnod**, picture him with a bald mother, a breastless mother, without a mother, and fall to the floor and weep.

[*five*]

Choices

A FEW DAYS later, the nurse insists on wheeling me into Radiology for the pre-op needle localization. I detest this idea, not only because I don't need a wheelchair, don't feel sick or weak, still don't actually believe I'm here for surgery, am waiting for someone to announce over the loudspeaker that this is all a big mistake. But also because Mike is a radiologist in *this* Radiology department. I've walked these halls numerous times over the past decade, carting babies and toddlers and resentment, barely registering the patients I flew past, the patients I sometimes envied because they commanded more of Mike's time and attention than the children and I did.

And while I've spent years waiting for him to be more husband and father and less "doctor," now I'm hoping I have everyone's undivided attention, that they haven't fought with their spouses, don't have some kid's recital they need to rush to, aren't making grocery lists in their head. I want to call a presurgical conference reminding them to think about me, concentrate on me, heal me, cure me, save me. When does the part where I become a bigger person kick in?

"A little cold," the technician says, hoisting my right breast onto the Plexiglas tray, while I sit in a chair. "You're lucky you have such large ones," she says. "It must have made nursing easier." She gestures to her nearly nonexistent chest, unwraps and holds up a long skinny needle with a hook and poings the end. "This is what we use so the surgeon knows *exactly* where to cut."

I nod, watch her manipulate my flesh, swab and mark it, and think how my breast doesn't even seem like a breast, like when I was nursing and the idea of breasts as sexual objects seemed absurd. I loved nursing and I was good at it; I always had plenty of milk—enough milk to feed the neighborhood, Mike and I always joked. I remember the contented look on each of my baby's faces, the nipple spilling from their lips—still moving, still suckling in their sleep. I felt so useful then, so powerful and competent, irreplaceable and absolutely amazed that I could nourish and comfort another human being with the milk my body produced, the warmth of my skin. . . . *Betrayer!* I want to scream at my breast. How could you? How could you? The words I would have used on my husband and his lover. The one he'll be afraid to take now that I am his sick wife.

The technician wrenches my flesh away from my chest wall and says to the nurse, "The best part about the Mediterranean was the topless beaches."

"You went topless?" the nurse asks.

"Hell yes," she says to the nurse. "There is no self-consciousness. And I figured when in Rome. . . . "

"Don't breathe," she says to me as the machine compresses my breast.

I think about my trip to Nice with Mike this past fall. Our first extended time away from the children in seventeen years, my second trip out of North America ever, and I couldn't relax, felt guilty the entire time, thinking it too extravagant, wrong to leave the children for such self-indulgent travel. As I sunbathed face down, Mike undid the top of my tankini, and when I sat up and my top fell away, I gasped and cupped my breasts with my hands and said, "I'm too old for this."

"No you're not." He tugged at my hands, wiggled a playful finger toward my nipple.

"It's just not my kind of thing." I fumbled with my straps.

"Your choice," he said as if I were obviously making the wrong one.

Now, with my breast smashed on a tray like a slab of meat, soon to be anesthetized and sliced open, excised and cauterized, sent to pathology to be cut up in a petri dish and analyzed, I wonder, Why hadn't I seized the opportunity? Why had I hesitated, cared what others thought, been so self-conscious, not relaxed more, celebrated every goddamned nanosecond of my life?

Brad Stevens, another radiology partner, whose wife was diagnosed with breast cancer a few years ago, walks in and over to the viewbox where he stares at both my old and new films from today. I see the tension pull his crisp white surgical jacket too taut against his shoulder blades as he says, "A couple more suspicious areas." Now Mike joins him and he's staring at the films too, raking his fingers through his hair as he says to his partner, "Are you thinking we should biopsy those areas?" Nancy, my surgeon (whose mother had breast cancer and worries about her own risk, something she revealed to me when I asked her preoperatively about prophylactic removal of my breasts and she said she wasn't unbiased because she'd contemplated it for herself), enters the room, nods at me, and then stands next to Mike and studies my films.

They both look at Mike and he says, "I don't think I should be involved in this. . . . "

"You're already involved," Brad says, his voice more clipped than I want it to be, making me all too aware of how much is being juggled in this pre-op room. All of their professional opinions, their egos, their personal brushes with breast cancer, their relationships with one another and me, the fact that they know that I know they're human, flawed, and that medicine is more primitive, less precise than most people realize. I picture the screen door Mike hung last spring, off by more than an inch in the door jam, rattling in the wind.

"You make all of us nervous," the technician says and pats my hand.

"Doctors' wives," the nurse concurs and rolls her eyes.

After everyone agrees that I, in fact, do harbor more suspicion, and as they bustle around me, numbing and needling and smashing my flesh in the way I imagine Mike handled the cadaver he dissected in medical school, the one that made him vomit the first day he came home from Gross Anatomy and tried to eat grilled chicken breasts with a white wine reduction sauce, I think: What an odd thing; a breast, a glob of fat and tissue that hangs off the front of your body, that changes from sexual to nurturing and back again, that requires special equipment, pushed up for dress up, bound for running, swabbed with betadine, tattooed with permanent marker, pierced with fishing hooks in four places before a lumpectomy.

"You have the most pre-op needles I've ever seen," the technician says, all of us gazing at my hideous pincushioned flesh.

"Is there an award for that?" I say, before the implication of all those needles sinks in. "Do they want to take my . . . " I whisper to Mike, my throat closing before "breast," and it strikes me that I'll never go topless in Nice. Never be a stripper. Never pose for *Playboy*. And now I want those choices back.

"No," Mike says and chuckles nervously and pats my head. "This is just precautionary," he says, referring to the additional biopsies they now want to take of the other suspicious areas. "So you don't have to wait for more cores after you heal from surgery. This way we'll know sooner. . . . "

I look to my surgeon whose lips are pursed before she says, "If it's diffuse DCIS that *is* what we'll do."

I swallow hard, say, "It's okay. I nursed my babies. They've served their purpose . . . it doesn't matter. . . . " Choke, sputter, heave and cry, in spite of my best efforts not to, as I realize it *does* matter, how much the idea of losing my breast, my choices, my life, horrifies me.

And that horror stays with me all the way down the long corridor, the four wiry antennas poking out of my chest, bobbing into one another. Now I understand why I'm in a wheelchair. I'm already physically and emotionally spent, and I might not willingly cross the threshold into the surgical suite otherwise. At the door, Mike bends down to kiss me, and I smell fear in the parched space between our lips—sour and brittle, laced with all the things we forgot to say, all the times we didn't love one another enough. I feel his effort not to tremble against my moist face, not to look grim as he mouths "BBBSS." Our private acronym: the one we carved into a wooden table at Chumley's in New York City our first year in love; the one both of us have traced on the other's back, over the years, when we couldn't sleep, after we fought, when there were no more words. Our code that means at turns: I'm sorry; please don't hold a grudge; I remember when; I love you. I mouth the letters back and our fingertips brush one last time before the nurse pushes me through the double doors toward the sterile bed prepared for me, and I have a vivid flash of me not waking up. But I worry more for him. Waiting is the harder gig.

six

Baby Doll

IWAKE TO the sound of my raspy-voiced neighbor flirting with the post-op nurse: "Make mine a double, darlin.'"

"A double what?" the nurse says and giggles and flips her stiff blond bangs out of her eyes and dust particles rise and fall, rippling through my groggy drift . . . her bangs bouncing off her forehead rhythmically . . . flip, flip, flip . . . she's still flipping toward him, when she pokes her head behind the wispy curtain and says, "You plan on joining us?"

I should say something, something witty, something wise, something memorable, something that will cement me here in this life forever. But all I can think is, I'll never be able to compete with him. For one thing, he's a man and she's a woman and . . . and now I've lost that train of thought . . . and another thing, I'm weak, awake from the anesthesia, but barely, in and out and out and out. *Come back,* I tell myself. *Come back.* This world is good, sprinkled with teeny tiny dust particles that flounce and float and waltz through the air, landing on my knuckle . . .

. . . the warm sticky tug of four-year-old Anna and three-year-old Maddy dragging me down the basement stairs, saying, "Baby Doll. Mommy, play Baby Doll." And me following in their determined footsteps. Down, down, down the creaky stairs to the cinder-block playroom that I'd set up with magical wands and pixie dust, a pretend corner that morphed from diner to castle to emergency room to pirate ship. Where I was an astronaut and Anna was She-Ra and Maddy a king, and all of us were chased by a near-sighted rhinoceros. Where I could be the kind of mother who not only played with her children but *wanted* to play with her children. A playroom where I could mother them and myself.

And I did, but Baby Doll snuck up on me. Baby Doll threw me. I hated Baby Doll. Cringed at the mere mention of Baby Doll because Baby Doll meant that I had to be Mary Poppins, while my girls pretended to march for Women's Rights, went to graduate school, out to lunch, to very important meetings. And while I encouraged and admired their choices, I was left holding the baby, burping and feeding and changing diapers. I was left cleaning and singing the baby to sleep while they did all the things I wasn't doing. Even though I was only in my early thirties and all of my friends were still single and traveling and building careers, amassing lovers and experiences while Mike worked 120 hours a week and we had no money for babysitters, no family nearby to help. And day after day, hour after hour, the boundaries between the girls' needs and mine blurred in that airless basement playroom, playing Baby Doll because I didn't know how to say no, felt as if saying no to them was like saying no to me.

But I was only going through the motions, thinking about other things in my head: how I'd ended up a full-time mother when I'd meant to work; how powerless I felt not working; how lonely marriage could be; how terrified I was of shouldering the monumental responsibility of not irrevocably screwing them up. I'd imagine them on a therapist's couch at forty saying, "My mother was BORED with Baby Doll." And when Anna returned from her "very important meeting," I was still holding the baby, but so absentmindedly that she was flipped upside down, her eyes lolling back in her head. Anna would climb on my lap and I wanted her to see how bad I was at Baby Doll and give me a break; but, no, instead she would cup my face in her sturdy hands and say, "More Mommy More." And that was the other thing about Baby Doll. There was always more and I was never enough. There wasn't enough *of* me, wasn't enough *for* me. Baby Doll and too many hours in the playroom and my mind turning to mush and me yearning to flirt and eat exotic mushrooms and go to Bora Bora and finish my graduate degree, finish one complete thought, write something, anything other than another grocery list, and go to the bathroom without someone trailing behind me saying, "Play Baby Doll, Mommy."

And now I wonder. . . .

Did I play enough Baby Doll? Too much Baby Doll? Should I have spent more time on my career? Gone to China with that grad school professor when I had a chance? Been more of a force in my own life? How do you know when you're immersed in endless days melding into one another that time isn't endless? In fact, it's so fleeting that everything you did or didn't do takes on monstrously exaggerated rhinocerific proportions when you're in a hospital recovery bed making tabulations: 45-and-a-half years times 365 minus 347 nonstop days of Baby Doll and countless hours of nursing and weaning and tantrums and cuddling and whining and Eskimo kisses and boo-boos and Band-Aids and shoelace-tying lessons and middle school traumas and orthodontia and soccer and Little League and basketball and first-love heartaches and college applications and two unsold novels and a couple of handfuls of publications and an abandoned graduate degree and 19-and-a-half years of a great big messy work-in-progress marriage on which the jury is *still* out and an old bureau at the top of the stairs crammed with mismatched socks. Where is Mary Poppins with her magic measuring tape telling me how I measure up?

"Decided to join us, huh?" I hear the nurse say.

"Sex on the Beach!" Raspy Voice shouts. "*That's* the name of the drink I was thinking of. I'll take a double one of those."

Giggling . . . giggling. . . .

Join them? Do I? Want to? I do . . . but . . . the peace between the breaths lures me. . . . I hear rubber shoes clutch and unclutch linoleum, stiff cart wheels whine, sense a thrumming so deep inside it feels as if someone is playing my nerve endings like a classical guitar. It aches but it feels. I. Want. To. Feel. . . . I want to come back. . . . I rub my eyes . . . see blurry pods of artificial light, a sea-foam blanket shrouding me, the tip of my nose. I run my tongue on the roof of my mouth. It's dry. I'm thirsty . . . part my lips . . . say, "I've made Sex on the Beach."

Laughter. Loud and raucous and real.

"The drink, I mean. I was a bartender once."

"That's what they all say," my neighbor snorts.

And the nurse bats her eyes, flips her bangs, flip, flip, flip, and I realize I'm back. I've made it through the surgery. Made my nurse and my neighbor laugh. But I also realize I can't change Baby Doll. The girls are grown and I have to make peace with what I did, what I didn't do. And I need more time, to launch my children and myself, to sort through and repair my shortcomings as a mother and a woman and a wife. I'm not ready to make the final tabulation, not ready to leave the party. I want to know what happens next: how my children turn out, whether I make something more of myself and whether that matters, whether Mike and I figure out how to be married. I want to know if my nurse and my neighbor hook up. I want to feel my breath tickle the tiny hairs that line my nose, to witness one spectacularly graceful dust oracle soaring through the air on the power of my exhalation.

seven

The Builders Come and Go

THE BUILDERS STAND at the front door talking of framing windows on the writer's hut that Mike surprised me with on my forty-fifth birthday last year. A sweet and overly generous gesture that makes me feel like a loser, as if a room of my own could redeem my years of mostly fruitless toil, as if there is enough time for me to waste on the page. *"There will be time, there will be time . . . time for you and time for me . . . time for a hundred indecisions . . . for a hundred visions and revisions."*

"Is it her birthday?" the foreman says from the front door.

"The flowers?" Mike says. "No. She had surgery yesterday."

Flowers. Flowers. Flowers everywhere! Shocking pink gerbera daisies, heavy blue heads of hydrangeas, a mass of daffodils in a yellow so optimistic I want to say *no, no, please don't pressure me that way,* insistent stalks of purple lily peaks with the card: *Let's Get Together Soon.* I sip coffee, read the paper, watch the builders come and go.

I noticed the little boy first—a vibrant redhead with a smattering of freckles and a heartbreaking, toothless grin. He held the door for me when I stumbled into gymnastics, a couple of months after we arrived in Madison, Alex fussing in my arms, until he saw the boy smile at him. The mother, Linda, had the same sweet smile, and lovely long fingers, when she patted me over to the chair beside hers. I told her we'd moved from Vermont. She told me she'd lived in Madison her whole life and that she was a painter, and when she spoke her fingers waved and fluttered like butterfly wings. And every week, through the entire session, while the girls jumped and flipped and twirled and the little boy, Olly, entertained Alex, we talked kids and husbands and running and yoga and art and poetry, about how hard it was to mother and create, how after the kids were grown we'd have more time . . . "*in a minute there is time . . . time for all the works and days of hands . . . "* and when the session ended we hugged and said, "Let's get together for lunch sometime."

But we didn't and time passed and then our daughters were in a summer drama class together and the teacher announced we'd have to make our own costumes. Anna was a rib eye (that *did* destroy her interest in acting), and I panicked (thinking I had no clue how to make her look like a piece of meat). But Linda turned to me and grabbed my wrists and said, "Don't worry, I'll help you." And she did. She made Anna look like the best damn rib eye in all of Wisconsin (something involving brown felt and stuffed nylons), and when the drama ended we hugged and said, "Let's get together soon." But we didn't. And after that I'd see her at the grocery store, at yoga, on the running trail, at the farmer's market and we'd smile and sometimes even clasp hands and say, "I'll call you." Her firm grip convincing me we would.

And then a few years ago, we saw her while out to dinner, her family in the booth right next to ours, Olly bigger, with a mouth full of braces and bands, but still a hint of that same sweet little-boy smile, and Linda and I smiled at each other and joked about the fact that we always said, "Let's get together." We both insisted we really meant it this time and this year we would. In the car on the way home I told Mike, "I *really* like her. This time I really *am* going to call her." And then a few months later, I was sipping coffee, reading the morning paper, leafing past the obituaries (not a section I usually read), but I paused because I thought, That woman kind of looks like Linda; then I read the words and it *was* Linda. She'd died, of ovarian cancer, and her funeral was the next day. . . .

"Why are you reading the obituaries?" Mike says now, setting a basket of blood-red tulips laced in baby's breath at my elbow.

"Remember Linda?" I say, biting my lower lip.

"Linda O'Malley?"

I nod.

"She died a couple of years ago," he says and places his hand over mine.

"I know," I say. "She had . . . the most beautiful fingers. . . . Did I ever tell you that?"

"I think you did," he says, his voice catching, too, as he folds up the paper and pulls me up.

"Why didn't I ever have lunch with her?" I ask, as if there's an answer that would change what was.

"I don't know," he says leading me over to the couch where we cuddle under a crushed-velvet throw, hold hands, wait for the call from the hospital, watch the builders come and go.

eight

The Call

THE HOURS PRESS in, sinking our bodies so deeply into each other and the worn squishy cushion, as we wait for the call, and it feels as if our family room sofa might swallow us into the coiled innards where Cheerio crumbs and sticky, loose change lurks. Waiting. Waiting. I've never been very good at waiting. Waiting for my mother to be the mother I wanted her to be caused me to grow up too fast, mature too slowly. Waiting to go into labor with each of my children resulted in two-week delays and pitocin. Waiting for the kids to grow and Mike to come home from the hospital paralyzed my ambition, while I told myself that time spent waiting was nothing in the scope of my very long life. Time was my most expendable commodity, plump with possibilities for me—later, when I'd work out my problems with Mike, with my mother, heal all my childhood wounds and finally figure out who or what I meant to be. Now later has arrived, and as Mike and I stare out the window at the cool February sky lording over gaunt branches and dry fisted leaves, I wonder how many more years I'll see the peonies bloom.

When the phone doesn't ring, I imagine all the biopsied areas are cancerous and it spreads and . . . I become a pothead because why the hell not? I'll call my old pot connection from college and order the best. I'll get a giant purple bong and spend my days with my head floating in pillows of bong smoke, except I hate smoke. Smoke hurts my throat, which is why I was never *much* of a pot smoker in college. So I'll move to California instead and go to one of those bakeries for medically sanctioned users, like the one I saw on *Weeds,* and Mary Louise Parker and I will become best friends. I really like her. She's so down to earth and real and honest, except for the whole drug-dealing thing. But I'll help her find a better guy and do something about that brother who's driving her crazy. And when my hair falls out, she'll help me find a Farrah Fawcett wig. Finally, the hair I wanted in seventh grade. Hair that can't be mussed at night and saves me time in the morning—maybe this isn't so bad. Me stoned with good hair. And then I picture my children and I ache for what I've done and can't undo. Maddy not even bothering me with her fashion show the night before the surgery, bringing me warm peppermint tea instead. The kind I make for *her.* Anna kissing and hugging *me* goodnight. Their stricken looks when they left for school this morning. Alex asking, "*When* can you play hoops with me?" Averting his gaze when I try to say *soon* and my eyes well instead. Reminding me of the forced role reversal with my own mother after her first nervous breakdown, the one thing I vowed I would *never* impose on my own children. How dare my mutated cells cause me to break that vow, how dare they disrupt the carefree business of my children's lives, steal their comfort, their belief in me.

I picture my friend Allison and remember feeling the dark shadow of a phantom limb following her everywhere and *her* mother died of cancer when she was twenty-something. Oh God, will I be my children's phantom limb? Am I their dark shadow? And who will know which kind of chocolate-covered raisins to pack in Anna's care package for college? That you can buy them only at the co-op on the east side of town and only when they're fresh (you have to ask the grocery clerk *when* they come in). Otherwise, the coating is too crackly and the raisins too stiff.

And Mike. What will happen to Mike? On our sixteenth anniversary at Tom's Burned Down Café on Madeline Island, Crazy Susan, who'd been married more times than Elizabeth Taylor and was very drunk that night, kept toasting to: "The couple who would rock in the rocking chair together and be able to say, I remember when. . . . " Who's going to rock in that rocking chair next to Mike when he grows old without me? He needs a companion. Someone who will love the children . . . like . . . like Rita, my yoga instructor. She's still single, and she's insightful and warm hearted with a head full of gorgeous stubborn curls. She's also tattooed and pierced and so solid and comfortable in her Voluptuous Goddess Body that she makes you want to be less afraid of who you are. She doesn't have any children of her own and she'd probably loosen Mike up in all the ways I haven't been able to. I picture her getting him into a Downward Facing Dog, talking him into a matching tattoo. I see them romping barefoot on a tropical island with the children, all of them happier without me . . . when the phone startles me.

Mike answers before the end of the first ring. His face doesn't look good. My stomach churns. I don't want them romping. I don't want them happier without me. I don't want to be a pothead.

"Your mother," Mike mouths. "Will do, Miriam," he says and hands me the phone.

"Hi, honey," she says. Her "honey" making me seven and her serving me Campbell's Chicken-with-Stars soup and Saltines on a TV tray, letting me watch *I Love Lucy* reruns. Maybe her voice can soothe this all away from Ohio.

She sniffles and stammers, says, "It isn't fair. You *chose* life. . . . " But I'm not seven and she isn't that mother anymore. Nothing she can say will make this go away. And I know that she's thinking about Daniel, my older brother who killed himself more than twenty years ago, whose death made such an indelible mark on my life that, still, every day, I go over the details. The line of miniature juice cans, the pill bottle, the car fumes. Details I know so well, not because I found him but because I feel guilty that I wasn't there, didn't know to be there, had fled to New York City to get away from all the craziness.

My mother sighs and I feel how hard it is for her to think about Daniel and worry about me. The too-much-ness of it all. And I know how much she loved Daniel, loves my sister, my other brother, loves me, deeply, hysterically, more intensely than anyone before Mike. Our connection so close at times, it felt as if she felt we shared one body, one mind. Except when she withdrew—and I felt lost and liberated.

"It's just so ironic." She interrupts my thought. My mother taught me irony and we both loved finding it in literature and in life. Except when it hit too close to home.

Ironically, I have waited and wished for the moment my mother would be willing to finally discuss the undiscussable. But not now. Now, I can't think about the ten tiny Mott's cans and their little silvery lids, the desperate thoughts that must have been running through my brother's head before he swallowed the pills, turned the key and how it must have felt for her to lose a child, I want to say that—that and more—so much more but not right now.

"Thanks for calling, Mom," I say instead, my voice hovering and then cracking over "Mom" as I hand the phone back to Mike and press my lips so tightly together I feel teeth marks denting my gums.

Before Mike hangs up and after he says, "We'll be in touch . . . as soon as we know," I hear the echo of her voice: "We have to work on our communication . . . get rid of the negativity. . . . "

We cradle the silent phone in the space between our laps, and I tuck my head into Mike's chest. We hold hands and stare at the impenetrable sky, and he hugs me closer . . . when the phone rings again.

This time Mike's anxious expression softens as he says, "Uh-huh. Uh-huh." Gives me a thumbs-up.

A thumbs-up? Thumbs-up must be good. And I'm up shouting, "Really? Really? I'm okay? Are you sure?"

He nods and motions for me to sit back down next to him.

"Thank you. Yes. Thank you," he says and hangs up the phone. "All the samples are negative," he says.

"Negative? Really? How negative?"

"Negative," he says, his impatience with my medical ignorance creeping back into his tone.

"Are you sure?" I ask anyway.

"I'm sure." He motions to me again and pats the space beside him.

"No chemo?"

He shakes his head. "They said they got clean margins—so probably no chemo."

"Radiation?"

"I'm not sure about the radiation. We'll discuss that with the oncologist."

"Oncologist? What do you mean oncologist? I don't like that word. . . . "

"You've had cancer, honey," he says and I'm a little annoyed that he feels he has to remind me.

"But it's out," I tell him.

"We got it out." He nods.

And I'm jumping up and down like a five-year-old, throwing my arms through the air and romping through the family room. I will romp the beach, make us happier, send Anna care packages, make tea, shoot hoops. I glance at the couch, see Mike schlumping, and I'm confused until my eyes land on the indentation where my body has left an empty space beside him—and it occurs to me that the last time we sat so close for so long, uninterrupted, was the first year we dated. Every day after we taught high school in Hell's Kitchen, we'd cuddle on my old ratty foam sofa, both of us happy to waste time with one another. I never felt more loved, more sure that this was the body I wanted next to mine. By the following year, there was medical school and soon after that babies and bills and too many chores and not enough sleep, so much wedged between us—until now, until this. And I think about this past week: how eagerly he filled my water glass; how tenderly he plumped my pillows; how content he seemed to be by my side.

"I feel as if I've lost my job," he says.

And I'm blown away by his self-reflection and honesty. But I'm also alarmed. I feel his need to be needed fighting my need not to have to need.

"I don't want to be your job. I want to be your partner. And I want to be healthy."

"I want you to be healthy, too," he snaps.

"I know that," I say and glance out the window and think, I've got issues to work out with Mike *and* with my mother, but now I have more time than I thought I did just minutes ago. The clouds shift, the tips of the branches stretch out and up, emboldening against the sky, and I believe in the possibility of possibilities once again.

I bend over and pull Mike up and into my arms. "I'm okay," I say to reassure both of us.

He nods and we collapse into two decades of embracing. Comfort trumping constraint. Then we're romping, into the kitchen, over to the refrigerator, rooting around for that old, cheap champagne tucked behind the leftovers. And when we find it, I pop it open, shooting the cork into the family room, the bubbles and froth cascading all over our hands as we share swigs straight from the overflowing rim.

[*nine*]

The Holiday Party

THE BURNT-ORANGE, harvest-yellow, and green Frank Lloyd Wright wave-inspired spherical carpet path leading to the room of banquet tables dressed in crisp white linens, strewn with confetti and miniature dessert-tier centerpieces, looks exactly the same as last year and the year before when we attended the Lakeview annual After-the-Holiday Holiday Party. Everything is the same—including the waiters setting up trays of pale chicken breasts and limp green beans and the huddles of people balancing wine glasses and

canapés against the low symphonic hum of overly polite chitchat.

Everything is the same—except me. I'm different. A
week post-surgery and I'm still exhausted, still sore,
still bruised, still afraid to look at my chest, so tender
inside and out that I tiptoe around myself as if the me I
always knew has been replaced by a stranger. I feel
some essence of me inside but it's buried pretty deeply
under skin that puckers and pulls in weird places. Like
that one-piece cotton gym suit from sixth grade. Only I
can't take this off and stuff it in the back of my locker at
the end of the period, vowing never to put it on again.

I know I shouldn't feel this way. I should feel better.
Happy. Relieved. It could have been so much worse. It
was small, noninvasive, they got it all. I'm fine, I'm fine,
I'm fine. This is the mantra I chant to myself repeatedly. And I do feel this incredible surge of love and
gratitude and joy for . . . my coffee, for . . . signing field
trip notices and searching for overdue library books
and sock pairs, duties that feel like a privilege now. And
snowflakes—who designed *that* precipitory miracle?
But all this aliveness is exhausting, and then BOOM
this wave of How-did-this-happen-and-if-I-don't-
know-how-will-I-prevent-it-from-happening-again
crashes in out of who knows where, knocking me sideways, buckling my knees. Like it does right now, as I
wobble over the polka-dotted carpet as we enter the
Holiday Party.

"I'm not sure I can do this," I whisper to Mike as I spot Brad Evans and his wife near the bar; my surgeon, Nancy, at the coat rack; Henry, who read my mammogram, and Pete, who performed the core biopsy; and half a dozen other people who last saw me topless and betadined and weeping in fear. Why am I here? This morning after I showered, I stared at myself in the mirror and decided if I could get my hair to fall in soft waves around my still unsettled face, I would go. And when I couldn't get it to look that way, I thought, I have to go anyway because if I don't, people will wonder and worry. And I don't want that. I have to show everyone that I survived: that I am still me; that I can eat chicken and dance.

"We'll leave as soon as you say so," Mike whispers back now and lets go of me and heads to the bar. Leaving me unarmed, unanchored, unglued.

"How *are* you?" Eleanor says. Eleanor: perfect mother, perfect doctor's wife. The kind of woman who exudes pure unyielding authority in all the areas that require authority. Making me wonder when or if I will ever reach that point of grown-up-ness. Her square jaw, her patrician nose, the impassive set of her alarmingly blue eyes, her smooth cap of honey-colored hair as consistently consistent as a mannequin's, provoking me to try to imagine one expression I could wear on *my* face and getting dizzy with the kaleidoscopic facial changes that effort wreaks. Her house: a page out of *Architectural*

Digest with lighted oil paintings and coordinating fresh-flower arrangements and oriental rugs (the fringe combed smooth with a special oriental rug comb, which I had no idea existed until she showed me) and decorative pillows in circles and squares and tubular shapes, in silk and Italian tapestry and made to look as if they were tousled just so, and no visible signs of ongoing life.

The first time we invited her and Stan over for dinner, soon after we moved to Madison, I walked from room to room with a giant box collecting old birthday party grab bags, plastic Happy Meal toys, Barbie high heels and then spent hours preparing miniature quiches, all sorts of stuffed things, and a dizzying array of hand-dipped chocolate-covered fruit to top the French tart to prove—what? That I could dip fruit? And all through dinner I nodded through Eleanor's tips on how to get your children into the Ivy League (which she had managed to do with *both* of her children). "Keep them focused. Emily [her oldest] loved animals so we told her, 'Be a veterinarian,' and sent her to veterinarian enrichment programs every summer and she had a four-page resumé by the time she graduated high school." I nodded as if I were taking mental notes, all the while knowing that the collage and glitter projects, the dancing to James Brown and hours of pretend and making up stories with my kids didn't qualify as focused. I didn't believe in micromanaging my children's future, nor tracking them at such a young age. I valued creativity and self-expression above resumé building. They were kids, for chrissakes, and having been a kid whose childhood had been cut short, I wasn't willing to sacrifice that for the Ivy League. Also, secretly, I believed my kids were so spectacular, so creative and bright and absolutely original, that they didn't have to follow those ridiculously limiting "getting into college" rules.

But, because I wanted her to think—what? . . . that I was like her? Wanted her to like me? I said, "We're thinking Dartmouth since that's Mike's alma mater." Truthfully, Mike was thinking Dartmouth. His undergraduate years had been the best years of his life (of course to me he would say the best years were after we met, but I know the truth). Dartmouth plucked him out of small-town Massachusetts and remolded and polished him into the man he thought he wanted and should be. I was thinking *not* Dartmouth. I'd attended grad school there while Mike was in medical school and had found the frat culture and anti-intellectualism and constant talk of prep school and the Hamptons stifling and uninspiring. Eleanor nodded approvingly. "Dartmouth is a *fine* school." "In Vermont we belonged to the science museum," I told her. "Anna and Maddy *loved* it!" This was true—they couldn't get enough of the bubble station. Then I stood to fetch the fruit-topped tart for Eleanor, when Maddy, who was seven then, and wearing that month's "uniform" (red feather boa, old pilly bathing suit and plastic heels, a smudge of pink frosting on her chin), clanked into the dining room and announced, "My Mommy sleeps with a pillow stuffed between her legs!"

"Fine! Great! Couldn't be better!" I say to Eleanor now at the Lakeview party, too loud and blushing all over again at the memory of Maddy. "They got it all out. Bouncing right back!" I nod my head as if it's a pompom cheering for me.

But when Eleanor looks at me, I know I am her worst nightmare, and I think this is the reason people like me should stay home: to not have to keep experiencing yourself as other people's dread; it is possibly the reason Brad Evans's wife "disappeared" for a few years after *her* diagnosis. Eleanor leans into me conspiratorially and says, "Well, that's a relief. You frightened all of us. We all said, if it could happen to you . . . so I *insisted* on an early mammo this year and thank God it was fine."

"Thank God," I say and chug half the glass of wine that Mike hands me before he walks away.

Then I smile at Eleanor and try to think of something else to say. Should I ask her about Emily's latest accomplishments? About their trip to Austria? Tell her that her hair looks . . . like it always does? I picture my mother making goofy faces up at me spying on her cocktail parties from the stairway rails and how she told me mindless chatter was a waste of words and breath. And then I think about Maddy and Anna rallying behind me as I got ready for the party.

"Fashion advice!" I'd yelled to the girls from my bedroom earlier that day. I'd been trying and retrying the black dress with the white trim that I'd bought for the party a month ago, *before* the surgery, *before* I knew I was going to have surgery. How odd to think that I had no clue that day at Banana Republic when I thought my biggest problem was whether I would find a dress for the party. And feeling relieved that I had found one that fit just right. And now for more than an hour, I'd pulled it on and off again so many times that my hair, which I'd spent all morning "doing," was an electric bay station, shocking me as I yanked the dress on again, when Maddy wandered in and threw herself on my comforter.

"See how it pulls over the swelling?" I said.

She swallowed a little too hard and I felt like an awful mother, for reminding her of the surgery, felt sorry for her because of me, wondered how and when we'd get beyond this.

She propped herself up on her elbows and said, "Put on a tighter bra."

That's when Anna tromped in, holding her black '40s-style vintage shoes out to me. "No matter what these always make me feel hot."

I slipped them on and even though they were a little tight and much higher than any shoe I'd ever worn, they arched my foot and tensed my calf so sexily, I forgot about the ill fit of the dress momentarily.

Maddy jumped up then and raised her index finger to indicate she'd be right back.

"Black tights," Anna said opening my sock drawer. "To elongate the leg."

"Here," Maddy said as she walked over to me and guided my arms through the sleeves of her black sweater, tying a knot over my chest. "Keep the shrug on all night."

"You're letting me borrow this?" This was the coveted piece of clothing that she and Anna had fought over a few weeks earlier. Maddy screaming, "Do not even *think* of touching that!"

Anna rolled her eyes at Maddy now and turned to me and said, "Be careful in the shoes. Sometimes the spiky heels catch on the carpet."

"And don't hunch," Maddy said.

I was touched and embarrassed by their indulgence. I didn't want them tiptoeing around me, didn't want to be this stranger who required special treatment. I wanted to snap out of this before the role reversal went too far and they became me and I became my mother.

I took a baby step toward them and the ground felt like sludge.

The girls giggled as my heel buckled.

"Maybe a little more practice," Anna said as the phone rang and they both jumped up.

"Remember, posture is everything," Maddy reminded me from the doorway. "You always tell us that!"

And I yelled, "Thanks, girls, and I promise I'll be back to my old self soon. . . . "

·   ·   ·

All at once I feel too hot with the pressure of trying to figure out the right thing to say to Eleanor. What to say? What to say? How's your Sub Zero? Sweat beading my chest, toes throbbing, wine pulsing through the veins. Too hot. Too hot. I wiggle off the shrug and my right boob throbs and another wave crashes in, side-swiping me and I sway and grab Eleanor's forearm.

"You okay?" she says as we both stare at my hand clutching her flesh. Am I okay? Okay? I'm not sure. I'm not sure of much of anything anymore other than I want to get out of here. But I nod anyway and let go of Eleanor, and she pretends to see someone across the room and politely slithers away.

I search for Mike in the sea of polished expressions, the symphony of chatter turning cacophonous and shrill, the walls moving in, and for a moment I forget what I'm looking for. And when I remember, still, I can't find him. I chug the rest of my wine and spot him cuffing Charlie Banks, chief of Orthopedic Surgery, on the shoulder and inching his way over to me.

When he reaches my side, I whisper, "Let's get out of here."

"How are you?" Charlie says to me.

"I'm fine!" I say. "And you?"

"Looking forward to dancing later," he says and winks at me. Mike pinches the back of my arm and mouths, *He doesn't know.* He doesn't know? Hmmm . . . I like that. Like that he's looking at the me from before. I smile at that thought, at Charlie. I glance over at the dance floor, picture myself last year, at the end of the night, my eyes closed, letting my body groove to the beat, and how in that moment I felt like my mojo was coming back. And now . . . now I don't recognize that woman who danced to "Love Shack," the one who bought this dress that's tugging on *my* chest, the one who threw her head back and laughed, really laughed, who didn't need special treatment, who thought Anna could go to college anywhere *she* wanted to, who never contemplated her own fragility. And my mojo? My mojo is so far gone I may never find it again. . . .

"No dancing," I say to Charlie. "I'm working on walking this year." I wiggle my heel.

Charlie laughs.

"And if you'll excuse us, we have to go now," I say and hook my arm through Mike's.

"They haven't served dinner yet," Charlie says.

"You can't make me eat that chicken *this* year!" I say, and Charlie laughs even harder now and I yank Mike's arm. But he doesn't budge. Instead he does his nervous chuckle-at-my-expense thing. I turn away and head toward the exit alone, feeling Mike's embarrassment cling to my back as I stride out of the party alone. But as the hum of small talk fades, my own internal voice strengthens and I tell myself that his embarrassment is *his* problem. In fact, all the fuss about these parties and me trying to impress Eleanor (who, quite frankly, is a more perfect person than I'll *ever* be), and my mother-in-law—who only wanted the best for her Golden Boy—and me trying to be the woman I thought he wanted and deserved, was all about him, what *he* cared about, and *my* problem was not being able to sift his feelings from mine. But I'm not willing to make that effort anymore. And I've lied to the girls. I'm not going back to my old self, the one who saw them through Eleanor's eyes—even for a second.

I want to go home and tell Maddy I'm glad she was and is my eccentric girl who speaks her mind and tell Anna that I hate Dartmouth for not recognizing how exceptional she is (even though I've told her that, I want to tell her again—*more* emphatically), that she's *better* than Dartmouth. Tell Alex I'm sorry I grew old when he was still so young. But I'll try to make it up to him, to all of them. And I am so relieved to see the exit that I pick up my pace and that's when my heel catches in a burnt-orange sphere (just like Anna warned me) and I'm stuck in the carpet. I yank and yank and when I still can't move, I think, Bring on the new me, puckery gym suit and all, and I yank my heel one more time, yank so hard I nearly topple from the sheer force of my will, and when it releases I trip in place and then steady myself . . . lift my heel and march straight toward the door, never once looking back, even though I don't have the keys to the car.

ten

Don't Blame Me for Your Cancer

O N THE WAY home from the party, Mike darts in and out of cars as if we're on a NASCAR race track while I clutch the dashboard and press my foot into my imaginary brake and say, "If I count the number of hours of doctor parties I didn't want to go to and divide it by—something—I probably could have written another couple of books."

"We're back to how my profession got in the way of your aspirations," he says, jerking the wheel around a nonexistent car and accelerating.

"And it's over with my agent," I say, thinking back to her recent e-mail suggesting we come up with a new concept for another novel. *The breast cancer thing is so gloomy. And maybe we could make the protagonist a little younger.* "She's sweet and all, and I know she did her best but I just don't think we have the same vision and my first book is essentially dead . . . " I say, admitting that for the first time to myself and feeling like such an idiot, thinking I might as well have been weaving baskets all this time. Why didn't I go to law school?

"Isn't it just like you to leave when the going gets tough?" Mike says and slams on the brakes, midway through the light. "No loyalty."

"What are you talking about?" I ask, my head bouncing against the headrest.

"Our marriage?" he says.

"I'm talking about my agent. . . . " Or am I? Now *I'm* confused. How much wine *did* I have?

"No wonder you aren't published," Mike says and floors the gas. "No stick-to-it-ive-ness. Is that what they taught you at your little experimental college?" Not so much wine that I don't recognize this well-treaded and famously unresolved fight. A fight that goes all the way back to our meeting in New York City, an unlikely match. His unwavering beeline into medicine underscoring my slightly more erratic career path: poet; advertising executive; actress; waitress; Yeshiva school teacher; waitress. Okay, mine wasn't exactly a path.

"Are we going to talk college now?" I say. "Because I have plenty to say about Dartmouth and you pressuring Anna into applying when we both knew it wasn't the right match. . . . "

"I'm not happy about that either," he says. And I know that's true. I know he thought he was doing the right thing, didn't expect her to be hurt by his good intentions. But that doesn't mean I don't harbor resentment about Dartmouth rejecting her and that I haven't gone over every little thing that happened from the moment we arrived in Hanover. Although I have to admit, at first I was enchanted with Dartmouth, too.

It was such a pretty place, both quaint *and* stately: the white-pillared Hanover Inn overlooking the Campus Green; the French restaurant in a turn-of-the-century yellow clapboard house, the very rootedness that permeated everything affiliated with the college. When Mike's friends came to visit for reunion weekends, I couldn't help but adore their undying loyalty to Dartmouth, to one another, couldn't help but admire the solid square of their shoulders, the certainty in the timbre of their voices, all that good-natured chuckling, all that slapping one another on the back, and me believing if I stood close enough their very essence would rub off on me.

But I soon discovered that I was too intense about the wrong things—too much poetry and philosophy, not enough tennis and tonics—and I didn't have the right clothes or the right body type. The Midwest, public high school, and my experimental college didn't make for the right credentials. But I didn't think it mattered. I figured with a few tweaks I could change all that. So I toned myself down, cut my hair into a neat bob, threw out the black vintage men's overcoat I'd scored on Canal Street, and squeezed my boobs into flowered Lanz dresses designed for flat-chested twelve-year-olds and learned the right names to drop. Sag Harbor—yes. Sylvania, Ohio—no.

But I would be wrong. By the time we left Hanover, more than a decade later, I still felt like an outsider, and had lost pieces of myself trying not to be.

"How do you think I feel?" Mike says now, his face twisting into a knot. I know this is hard on him. I know Dartmouth was good for *him* and he still can't fathom why it wouldn't be good for everyone, still doesn't believe it could have rejected his daughter. How do I think he feels? I think he feels torn and doesn't know what to do with that feeling. But before I can answer, the car weaves past the strip mall: Video Station; Cellular One; Subway; Dairy Queen; Supercuts and my boob aches. And I remember that we aren't in Hanover anymore and I've had surgery and this may be the longest stretch of time I've gone *not* thinking about *that* and I say, "I think you feel ambivalent and I'm wondering whether there might not have been a little overreaction in pre-op."

"What?"

"My surgery? Did they have to cut out golf ball–sized chunks of my flesh?" Even with the swelling I can feel indentations forming erratic impressions.

"Do you have to overanalyze everything?"

"Yes, I do. . . . That *is* something I learned at *my* little experimental college. . . . "

"Are you questioning my medical judgment?" he says, as if he's addressing the president of the Medical Ethics Committee.

"Not yours alone. Everyone involved. Think about it. The nurse talking about how doctors' wives make them nervous and. . . . "

"Doctor's wife? That's a *good* thing," he says, making a sharp right turn into our neighborhood, swerving a little too close to the curb.

I tumble against the door and say nothing.

"Do you know how many women would love to trade places with you?" he says, making a quick left at the "Welcome to Maplewood" sign. I try to summon that "life-is-so-precious-I-can't-get-over-the-miracle-of-a-snowflake" feeling as we ascend the hill, but it's gone, replaced by another fight so familiar, so relentlessly unresolved I might as well be having the fight with myself. The one where he's the catch and I'm the lucky catchee and I usually scream, "If you'd like to find a woman who would like to trade places with me, I wouldn't want to stop you!"

But I ignore his "rhetorical" question and continue with my train of thought. "And George's [the pathologist] and Brad's [the pre-op radiologist] wives both had breast cancer and so did Nancy's [the surgeon] mother. It crossed my mind for a moment in pre-op but the implication didn't sink in until now. . . . "

"It always comes back to this, doesn't it?" he says, approaching the blind corner halfway to the top. "You not respecting my profession."

While I am skeptical about his profession's ability to heal and/or diagnose all disease, and while his profession has eaten away at our marriage and our family life, and honestly, if I'd known how unprepared and ill suited I was for the 24/7 Doctor's Wife role, I never would have married a doctor. So he's right. But this isn't about that. This is about why he would rather defend his colleagues than try to understand what I'm saying. "This is a question of loyalties," I say, picturing him with his Dartmouth buds, his partners, his colleagues.

"I don't mind," he says, glancing at my chest. "Really. You're still beautiful to me and . . . who else is going to see it?"

Hmmm . . . I hadn't thought of someone *else* seeing it. I was stuck on *me* not wanting to see it. "That's not the point," I say. "It's my breast. . . . My breasts were one of my . . . best features . . . and now. . . . " I cup my smaller, permanently dented breast as the street lamps illuminate Mike's white-knuckled grip on the wheel and we pass the remodeled cape and its shiny stainless mailbox, the front stoop flanked with stone lions, the white-brick Georgian shrouded in weeping willows, the tile-roofed Tuscan with the brand-new hot tub, each house such an integral part of my daily landscape— the one that was so *boring,* so ongoing, the ongoingness so absolute and unequivocal—that I can't remember the last time I registered the details, making me wonder *how long I have been sleeping, how long I have been drifting alone through the night.*

"We did what looked like the right thing to do under the circumstances," he says and clears his throat. "Cancer is unpredictable and if it had been diffuse DCIS, we were looking at taking the breast anyway. Might it have been handled slightly differently? Perhaps. Might some fears have been projected onto your case? Possibly. Should we maybe have slowed down and—"

"If you ask and answer one more of your own questions I'm going to scream," I say and think, He's not being as nice to me as he was before and maybe that means nothing was ever wrong with me, maybe I imagined everything. . . .

"Don't blame me for your cancer," he says and slams on the brakes.

The word "cancer" stabs me, reminds me I'm not out of the woods. That there is no way out of the woods. I've had cancer. I have a serious medical history. I am at high risk for recurrence and while "they got it all out" my cells have proven that they aren't afraid to mutate. I am the woods. And if I wanted to cheat on Mike, which I never have, but am so mad at him, I'm thinking I might want to now . . . who would want a woman who'd had cancer? And it occurs to me that my butchered breast doesn't bother him because it brands me: UNDESIRABLE WOMAN. I swallow the last trickle of relief I'd been coveting since the news it wasn't invasive, and feel it churn inside.

As we approach the final turn at the moss-covered Tudor and onto our street's lampless, pitch-black cul de sac, I replay the scene in *Terms of Endearment* when Emma is in the hospital and she's saying goodbye to her sons, telling her older son that his hair is too long and that she loves him more than she loves herself and that she forgives him for pretending he doesn't love her and he's crying, and the little brother is crying and the mother is crying and by the time we pull into our driveway, I'm weeping into my fist.

eleven

Mother's
Little Helper

GIANT SHOE CLUMPS of tangled laces and open tongues crawl across the front hallway, cell phones sing and bleat, laughter wafts down from the attic, in from the family room and I'm thrilled. Thrilled that our daughters have their friends over, that they're having fun, that I'm here and not in the hospital. That the surgeon got it all out and I'm fine. I'm fine. I'm fine. But I don't want to be seen with my eyes red from crying, so I tiptoe upstairs to take a warm bath. As the water fills, I think about Mike and the party and our fight, our stupid, nasty fight that I'm too tired to ever resolve, open the medicine cabinet, see my Mother's Little Helpers, hear them sing that everything is different today.

In the tub, as warm water trickles over my toes, I try to figure everything out, to trace the origin, to pinpoint exactly when my cells decided to turn on me. . . . Was it the day I started my novel about the woman who finds the lump in her breast? Why did I write that book? Why did I wear it day after day like a too-tight wet t-shirt, writing so far into the book that I was the book and the book was me? Writing and weeping and forcing myself to feel what it might feel like to have cancer. Could a person write their own destiny?

Or was it when I'd nearly finished—and I wanted to feel relieved that I had another book my agent could sell, wanted to believe that this was the one that would finally justify the hours I'd spent writing, the times I hadn't made dinner, hadn't volunteered, said "no" to one of the kids' requests because I was "working"and I worried the novel might not be anything more than a series of words strung together like cheap snap-on beads? My nerves so rattled I couldn't sleep. (Maybe my agent *is* right, maybe nobody will care if the woman has breast cancer or not.) Am I talking about my book or myself?

Or was it the night after the nearly topless day in Nice and Mike and I were walking home from Old Town along the boardwalk and arguing about whether we should go to Paris a day early and Mike was pouting because we hadn't had enough sex and I wondered, How much sex is enough sex? Wondered why I didn't want to have more sex.

I thought about sex and I thought about wanting to have sex and sometimes when I saw Mike across a room—like at my friend Martha's fortieth Punk Rock birthday party and I'd gone early to help set up the dance floor and I glanced up and saw this sandy-haired guy wearing a tight black t-shirt and a dog collar and a killer grin and I felt myself flush when Martha said, "That's your husband."

My husband? Mike? Preppy Mike wearing that? It was like seeing him for the first time, or like seeing him as someone else, someone new. . . . But often the sex was payback, obligatory. I'd count up the days and the nice things he'd done and calculate the compensation. Blow jobs were the most valuable, roughly worth the equivalent of three quickies. Is a woman a whore if she has sex out of obligation even if it's with her husband? I'd asked myself and friends that countless times and still didn't know nineteen years and three kids into the gig.

If my book sold and I earned more money than Mike and *I* wanted to have sex and *he* didn't, would *he* be a whore? What were the rules? Where was the instruction book? And when exactly did we become a cliché—the frigid wife with the sex-starved husband? Although I didn't really *feel* frigid, I just didn't feel like having sex with my husband. On this trip. When we'd spent more time fighting than flirting. And this is what we were arguing about along the boardwalk in Nice. This and whether or not we should go to Paris a day early.

Only I didn't say that exactly. I said, "God is going to punish us for not appreciating how good we have it." But I didn't mean *I* wanted to be the lesson in appreciation. Do you hear me, God? I meant we were in France and all we had to worry about was whether to stay in Nice another day. Not to mention we had three healthy, smart, absolutely mind-bogglingly incredible children, enough money (finally) to travel, and there was a war in Iraq and poor beggar children on the streets of Nice, and soon (although of course I didn't know it) we would be faced with cancer.

Maybe it all went further back. My breast surgeon *did* say most cancers are decades in the making—and how does all this relate to the cancer? I'm not sure. But, I have felt toxins, toxins from my marriage, from my parents' marriage, from Mike's parents' marriage, from all the shitty marriages all over the world, penetrate my flesh. I shudder. Clutch my breasts, think, I'll run away because if I leave the house, the neighborhood, the state where I received the diagnosis, I can leave all of this behind. I'll go to New York City because I've lived there before and I remember how anonymous I felt in the city. Anonymity is good because if nobody knows this damaged me, then this me will not exist.

Then I picture running into an old boyfriend in Times Square. For some reason Times Square pops into my head. The neon lights, the porn shops, the flashing Broadway show signs, DREAMGIRLS DREAMGIRLS. And he (the old boyfriend) asks how I am and I feel compelled to tell him about my diagnosis and when I say the word "cancer," I burst into tears.

No, I need to go to a deserted place, a place I've never been to, an unmarked island where they've never heard of mammograms. Why did I marry a radiologist, anyway? A person always looking for what's wrong with the picture? Talk about bad karma. Mike's right. I *am* blaming him for my cancer. I am. I am. I am. I am the egg man. I am the walrus. Coo coo ca choo. I am too hot.

I hoist myself out of the tub and the room spins, twirls around me like Isadora Duncan. I am Isadora Duncan. I am a scarf. I am *her* scarf. I am flying. I feel light, lighter. . . . I am vapor. I'm nauseated. I really am sick. They were wrong about my diagnosis. It's much more serious. I'm dying. I gasp for air. I stumble toward the door, using the walls as crutches. I should call out for help, remember all the teenagers in the house, don't want to be the sick mother, don't want to stigmatize my children. "Mike, Mike, Mike," I say, my words sucking into black.

"Your head is bleeding, Mommy." Alex is standing over me.

"Your hair is too long and I love you more than I love myself," I mumble the lines from *Terms of Endearment*. . . .

"Huh?"

"I'm okay," I say. I'm alive . . . alive . . . alive. . . . How many lives does a person get? Sylvia Plath kept rising like Lazarus in spite of herself and I just used up two in the last week, this and the surgery, and there was the time I had pyelonephritis at five (I knew my parents were worried because they bought me three new Barbies *and* the deluxe carrying case), and I had an anaphylactic reaction to soft-shell crab at twelve, my throat closing as my mother rushed me to the ER. And when I was giving birth to Anna, the only reason I didn't die is because I said, "Boy, this is relaxing," and up until then I'd been screaming and choking Mike and he yelled at the nurse, "Check her blood pressure," and it was 60/0. And there was the time my mother-in-law gave me Benadryl for my runny eyes after I'd had a glass or two of wine and by the time I got home I couldn't open the car door. . . . I hope I'm a cat. Am I a cat? Why am I lying on my back in the hallway?

"Mommy? Mommy?" Alex looks afraid. "Dad?" he yells.

I push myself up. "I'm really okay, honey." I feel a little dizzy, but I'm fine. I'm fine. They got it all out. I'm fine. Fine fine fine fine fine fine fine fine.

Mike standing over me. "What the hell happened?"

"Nothing," I say. Use his body to leverage my body upright.

"You're bleeding." He points to my eyebrow.

"I'm fine," I say, again. A phrase I'm getting really tired of saying. If I really *were* fine I wouldn't have to keep saying it. Would I?

He leads me to the bed and stuffs pillows under my legs.

"Do you think it was my mother's little helper?" I slur. Giggle.

"You took one?"

I nod. Giggle some more.

"You know you can't mix those with alcohol," he says.

"If I knew that," I say, "then why would I have done it?" I make an L with my fingers pressed to my forehead. For LOSER.

Then I'm laughing and saying, "duhhhh." I'm not dying. I'm getting younger. I'm a teenager now. Laughing some more and he's pinching me and forcing water down my throat when all I want to do is close my eyes, take a little nap . . . sleep . . . dream about DREAM-GIRLS, my escape.

twelve

About the House
and the Fourth of July
and Turning Forty

O F COURSE THERE are no dreamgirls, no old boyfriend, no escape because this is a memoir. My life. And it's messy and complicated and gloomy (yes, possibly even gloomier than that damn breast cancer novel), and there isn't enough sex. Maybe I should sex it up a little bit.

But I don't. Not yet.

Instead, I wake with cotton mouth and the kind of ass-kicking hangover I can't remember having since my early twenties, a dull ache on the side of my head, and a vague memory of bathing and falling and crawling into bed. And on top of all that, I feel like I'm getting sick, which worries me because I *never* get sick (okay, except for the cancer thing, which I keep conveniently forgetting).

I wonder, Does that qualify as sick if I didn't *feel* sick? But, this morning, my throat is sore. Definitely sore and I'm not entirely convinced I want to get up, the act of lifting my head from my pillow, of trying to figure out how to let go of my old self and be The New Me, to remember what it is I *do* on a Sunday, seeming like *way* too much work. So I tuck the comforter under my chin and think about Mrs. Hart, the woman who lived in this house before me.

She died in bed, in *this* bedroom, of a cold turned to pneumonia fifteen years before we bought the house from her children after her husband died. All those years she was gone, he left the entire house—her collections of vegetable-patterned dishes, her tarnished silver platters, her etched glassware, her architectural artifacts, her jaunty clothes, her hats and dresses and silk-lined suits and gloves, her fifty-five-gallon vat of lye in the basement waiting for more furniture to strip—a shrine to her life, as if he were expecting her to walk through the door any minute.

Her stuff seemed of another era, another sensibility altogether. One that took belongings more seriously than I did. I'd always been skeptical of possessions, the lure and the trap of a consumer-driven, materialistic world and so while I didn't exactly eschew them, I didn't covet them either. I wasn't a "shopper," wasn't a "collector." I mistreated things, as if by mistreating them I lessened their appeal and their power. But Mrs. Hart's stuff made me see "things" differently, see *her* things as an expression of who she was. They told a story, that she cared about aesthetics, that she liked to get dressed up, celebrate life, have fun, party.

And she did. The entire backyard was wired for outdoor entertaining, with jerry-rigged speakers and lights in the trees and a giant old fountain from Richland Center town square. The gardens and patios paved with Old Chicago brick that the Harts hauled and hand laid into intimate terraces. And even in its weedy, overgrown day-lily-gone-wild state, I could imagine the Gatsby-esque soirées the Harts were rumored to have thrown. Every morning, according to legend, Mr. Hart had coffee and heated political talk with the neighbor from across the street.

And in an old cupboard in the basement we found a series of watercolors painted by the wife of the famous architect next door to the Harts' house from *her* house signed to Mr. Hart (Ed), making me wonder if she'd been in love with Ed. I have no real evidence of this. But I *do* know they lived larger than life, they were more colorful, more passionate, more fully engaged in the business of life than most people and when Mike and I first walked through the house, the walls literally crumbling down, we both felt a world that exuded life force kept in limbo since Mrs. Hart's death and we wanted to bring it back.

By the estate sale, just before the closing, Mrs. Hart's unclaimed clothes and dishes and knickknacks had been stripped from the closets, emptied from the shelves, a world artfully conceived over time; sorted, coded, and priced for sale. It seemed so clinical, so businesslike, so wrong that her "things" would be hauled away by strangers.

So we tried to buy as much of Mrs. Hart's stuff as we could (which wasn't that much since buying the house and renovating it were already beyond our still-in-debt-from-medical-school budget). But we ended up with the old pine dining room table and the wooden latched craft cupboard and the Oriental rug nobody wanted.

Standing in the middle of the dining room, as strangers pawed and haggled over her matching tomato plates, I vowed to make it up to her by filling her home with comfy furniture, books and art and music, and the smell of simmering soup and a dining room anchoring the hub with *her* pine table, big enough for the kids to do their homework and art projects and later to entertain all the fabulous, creative, fascinating people we would meet.

Up until we found the house, we'd had a bit of a rocky start in Madison. Both of us were hoping the

move would finally root us as a couple and a family—
with a baby and two young kids—thinking that since it
wasn't "home" to either of us, it would force us to make
"home" together. But it didn't feel right. Mike, having
never lived anywhere west of New York City, thought
Wisconsin was a foreign country. He was palpably
homesick. His New England slow-to-warm-up sensibility was widely interpreted as humorless and cold,
while he was widely skeptical of people smiling at him
for no apparent reason, asking him, "How you doing?"
then walking away before he could answer.

I reminded him that nobody spoke to me *at all* the
first year we moved to New England and he said, "But
when they did, they meant it." And even though I was
from the Midwest, Madison had its own culture and
not just the progressive one that had attracted us. It
had something to do with football, cheese, bratwurst,
and names of people and places we didn't know, and
the unspoken language and nuances every place pos-
sesses and requires new people to decode. It made me
homesick, too. Not for a particular place. But homesick
for the feeling of home. A kind of global homesickness
that made me acutely aware of transience and the
fact that I had moved too many times as a child and
that Mike and I had moved too many times (nine times
in the first twelve years of our marriage). Moving was
exhausting and not just the physical part of packing
and hauling and unpacking belongings. But the part

that called on brainpower for things like finding the bathroom in the middle of the night, jolting me from semiconsciousness into a forced life assessment. Which house? Which bed? What year? And ending in a full-blown existential crisis. Where am I? Where have I been? Where am I going? All just to pee.

I admit I made mistakes in Madison. I only skimmed the Village handbook (they called it a "Village" but it was really a planned community of just over 600 homes) that listed the names of the Village Officials, the Board of Trustees, more than two dozen Standing Committees and half a dozen Special Committees, and a full page devoted to the history of the Fourth of July:

"A day-long family celebration . . . starting with a challenge baseball game between the bachelors and the old married men . . . a bake sale sponsored by the Village League . . . the big children's parade . . . fire engine rides, balloons, Popsicles, carnival games, water fight, pie-eating contests . . . a picnic dinner on the school grounds . . . the climax of the day comes when the villagers gather at twilight at The Country Club for a spectacular fireworks display."

This was the kind of hyper-organized event that terrified me. I didn't know how to *do* suburbia, didn't belong in a place that handed out a handbook warning: *Every resident is REQUIRED to destroy all NOXIOUS WEEDS on their property.* How was I to know what was noxious? But as I said, I hadn't read the handbook carefully, so the morning of the Fourth, as I walked our dog and saw driveway after driveway filled with red, white, and blue bikes and flags and patriotic floats, I realized that all the children in the neighborhood, all the children in the country, the world, the universe for all I knew, decorated their bikes for The Parade.

I should have known this, I'd lived in America, was an American. But I'd never been very tuned in to the Fourth of July. I'd always viewed it as a way to force patriotism down people's throats, not to mention that fireworks reminded me of war. But, the fact is that on *this* particular Fourth, as I perused the new 'hood, I was convinced I would ruin my children's entire futures, cause them to turn to drugs and unprotected sex and technical college, by denying them decorative participation.

So as I rounded the top of the hill, approaching a driveway jam-packed with more streamers, flags, banners, and patriotic paraphernalia than anyone could possibly use in a lifetime, I introduced myself to The Mother, who was wearing a red, white, and blue dress and a matching star-studded visor and flag earrings (and *not* ironically), and asked her if I could borrow a few rolls of streamers.

She eyed me in my black running shorts, black running tank, and Black Dog baseball cap (pretty much my standard morning uniform then and now) and

said, "I guess . . . but next year you better be prepared."
She tossed me a few unraveling rolls.

It turned out she was one of *the* Queen Bees of the
Village—a person, I was later told, I shouldn't have ex-
posed my cluelessness to. It probably didn't help that
up until that point, I'd made only two friends: a Norwegian woman in Madison for her husband's sabbati-
cal year, whom I'd met at the ice skating hut and with
whom I'd walked every day that first winter. I taught
her English slang, while she taught me how to brace the
cold. And a Puerto Rican high school senior whose
mother had died of AIDS and had run away from
home to live with her boyfriend's family in Madison.
I'd hired her as a mother's helper so I could try to think
about starting to write again. But mostly we just talked.

And while I kept telling myself I was too old to try to
join this Maplewood Suburban Sorority or any sorority
(my college didn't even *have* sororities; I *hated* sororities), it was the third-grade girls at Anna's school who
bullied me into trying. Initially, the girls were attracted
to Anna because she was new but soon grew threatened
by her. The leader staged a conspiracy straight out of
Mean Girls, snapping Anna's pencil in half before a
math test while smiling at the teacher and threatening
not to invite her to her birthday party if Anna wouldn't
be her *dog,* tend to her every need and literally crawl
behind her on her hands and knees. This was years

before *Mean Girls* existed, before people were willing to admit that girls terrorized one another. When I spoke to Anna's teacher about it, she pooh-poohed me, said the girl in question was from one of the most established families in the neighborhood and would *never* do anything like that.

So for Anna's sake, for the sake of trying to fight third-grade social injustice, I volunteered for the May Day committee and went to coffees where educated women listened to the hostess discuss her method of rotating dinner plates once a week so they all got used—and aged—equally. And I failed. Failed to know how to respond to plate rotation. Failed to make my way into the neighborhood social groove. Failed to pave Anna's way in with those third-grade mean girls who stayed bitchy right through high school (who even today I have a hard time seeing without cringing). I guess I never recovered from my Fourth of July transgression and the subsequent rumors that I was from New York, quirky, "her own person," as if I shouldn't be.

So by the time we found this dilapidated house, I realized the only way to cure my and Mike's homesickness was to burrow our displaced roots into Mrs. Hart's sturdier ones and generate our own. I threw every bit of myself, everything I knew and believed, into restoring it.

Then I was turning forty. How that happened, I have *no* idea. *Before* it happened it seemed so remote I couldn't imagine the day ever arriving, and then once it *did,* I was incredulous. Last I knew I was twenty-eight. How did the years meld and blur?

On the last night of my thirties, Mike said, "I tried to throw you a surprise party, but none of your friends could make it."

Ouch. *That* hurt. And shook me. By then, my Norwegian and Puerto Rican girlfriends had both left Madison and the "friends" Mike was referring to were Allison, an old friend of mine from NYC who'd moved to Florida and whose husband had just run off with a twenty-five-year-old manicurist, leaving her with two small children to raise, and Glenda, my best friend from college, who had just relocated to Virginia and, between her three kids and her own difficult husband, said she couldn't make it either. I realized that I'd devoted so much of my time and energy to the house and the kids, and trying to make friends with the parents of *their* friends, that I didn't have any real friends myself. (Shortly after that I started hanging out with Martha and Rachel and my running buddies and my yoga girls.) But the night of my fortieth, after I felt good and sorry for my friendless-ass self, I told Mike I'd had it with moving. In fact, I told him I wasn't *ever* moving again, that they'd have to wheel me out of this house on a stretcher. . . .

They may have to wheel me out of bed, I think, now, as I rub my eyes and yawn and stretch and force myself to sit up and slide my legs off the bed and lug myself into the bathroom and examine the nasty cut and bruise on the edge of my eyebrow. I splash water on my face and run through my stats. I'm forty-five. I'm healthy. No. I'm forty-five. I've had breast cancer. My agent hates the book I spent the last year and a half on and hasn't been able to sell the one that took me the decade before to complete. I either have to find a new agent or a new profession.

I need a Plan B. Except I don't have a Plan B. I barely have a Plan A. I turn off the water and think, Well, at least I have my children. Then I remember, the girls dressing me for the party, Alex finding me passed out on the bathroom floor. (I have my children but do they have *me?*) And my marriage? My feelings about it change half a dozen times a day, from patting myself on the back for staying married and faithful for two decades, to thinking that's only because I'm a coward and isn't the truest test of love and marriage whether it can survive betrayal? And how can either of us figure any of this out now that I've complicated the equation? Which one of us would be brave enough to say uncle now? *Is that all there is?* My mother always played that Peggy Lee song while setting up cocktail parties, filling the Plexiglas ice bucket with cubes from our brand-new Frigidaire automatic ice maker. Peggy and my mother would hold the notes so long, so mournfully, I thought the song was about longing. But now, as the words run through my head, I wonder, literally, if this *is* all there is. Okay, so basically, I feel like shit. Shit shit shit shit shit. But I'm here. I'm alive. They got it all out. I'm lucky. I'm fine I'm fine I'm fine I'm fine I'm fine.

I dry my face and pull my hair into a ponytail. The clamor of pots and pans and the smell of Mike's banana-batter French toast and strong coffee nudge me into another day. Reminds me that this is what I love about life. All the physical sensations. The buttery feel of the worn wooden banister on my palm as I descend the stairs, the nicks on the wall that remind me of Alex dragging his favorite baseball bat up to bed, of the old desk we found in the back of the florist shop and talked the owner into selling and moved into Anna's room, of Maddy trampling up and down the stairs with her gaggle of friends, the anticipation of biting into warm French toast. If only my head wasn't throbbing and my throat didn't ache and I wasn't aware that acknowledging my love of all this only further intensifies my fear of losing it.

Downstairs, I find the girls at the dining room table doing homework and sipping tea. Alex is cuddled under a throw on the sofa in the family room, telling the girls, "Blood was spurting all over me."

"Not spurting," I say to the girls and touch my eyebrow.

"Eww. That looks nasty," Anna says.

"Don't you know you can't mix pills and booze, Mom?" Maddy says. "That's what killed that girl from Middleton."

"Enough," Mike says. "It was a mistake. Leave your mother alone." He pours me a cup of coffee.

I turn to Alex and say, "I'm sorry if I scared you."

"You didn't scare me," he says. "I knew you'd be okay. You're always okay."

I walk over and hug him, all of him, the sweet sour smell of unwashed hair and maple syrup and naiveté, his solid heft surprising me, and I feel my breath catch, glad he still sees me as "okay," immediately followed by my worry that I'll disappoint him.

I shuffle over to the girls and hug each of them and Anna says, "What time are we going to run today?"

"In an hour," Maddy says to Anna.

"That will give you time to digest," Anna says to me.

Now I remember, that's what I normally do on a Sunday morning. The girls and I run and later I take them to lunch and then (if Maddy doesn't have too much homework) she goes grocery shopping with me and I make a big Sunday-night dinner. But I can't run and I don't feel like shopping. In fact I really feel like going back to bed so I can wake up and start all over again. No head injury. No sore throat. No cancer threat. "Not today," I say. "Not yet. I have to get the okay from my surgeon next week before I can run, and I think I'm coming down with a cold."

"You *never* get sick," Alex says.

I nod and for half a second I believe the myth of me, that I never get sick, that I am strong and healthy, an ox, invincible, that I have defied age, that I will always be here . . . and when I remember that my cells have oxidized at a younger age than most, I feel like the fool on the hill.

Mike takes my hand and, without a word, leads me to the front hall where he points to my boots and guides my arms into my winter coat and then pulls me out the door. I follow him, tiptoeing over the icy upper driveway, crunching through the crusty snow and into the backyard, and he nods to the writer's hut, the windows and doors up and the stucco painted the same buttery yellow as our house and says, "Is this how you imagined it?"

This is his way of saying I'm sorry about our fight and I believe in you and your writing and the future. The future is where I choke. Honestly, I'm not sure I trust the future anymore. It doesn't exist until it happens and it doesn't happen if you don't exist. Well, I guess it happens whether you're there or not, it's just that you don't experience it. The hard truth is that at some point this world will go on without me. But the very thought of counting on the future or planning for it bewilders me.

And really, I shouldn't be surprised. This isn't the first time I've questioned the future. The first time was when my father left our family and my childhood was destroyed (with the family photos my mother cut my father's head out of). . . . And then my mother's first breakdown when I had to accept that she wasn't going to be the mother I'd known and I'd have to be a different kind of daughter for both of us to move forward. Then my brother's emotional collapse that made me question the concept of sanity. Each of those times I thought, *This* is the worst thing. It can't get any worse than this. And then . . . middle of the night . . . phone ringing ringing . . . my father's voice rising and cracking. "Your bro-ther killed himse," he sputtered, choked, and gulped, and in the awkward sighing and crackling connection, I realized I'd never heard my father cry, never felt him falter.

"How did it happen?" I asked over and over again as if something in the details could make it not so. I woke my sister and we huddled shoulder to shoulder that night, at the tiny kitchen table, lighting candles and cigarettes, melting wax over our trembling fingers, wiping tears from each other's eyes until the sun dared to rise.

A hazy year or so later, I met Mike. A button-down-collar guy who'd descended from earnest, puritanical people who taught him if you work hard and play by the rules you'll get what you want (while my family preached absurdity, debating *Waiting for Godot* for sport). And even though I didn't believe in or understand "the rules," I loved that he did. Loved that he was so unlike anyone I'd ever dated, that his world was cleaner and clearer, less sardonic, more sure than any I'd ever known. And it occurred to me that in deference to my brother, because *I'd* survived and *he* hadn't, I'd been treading water, but barely, and—corny though it may sound—Mike was my raft.

Mike is looking at me so expectantly now, waiting for my answer. *Is this how I imagined it?* Did I imagine that I would discover that behind the white colonial facade, in spite of following "the rules," his family was as screwy as my own (comforting and confounding me equally) and that he *hadn't* been the raft, that he'd needed a raft, too, and we'd nearly drowned one another trying to hang on?

I run through *What Ifs* in my head. If I hadn't married Mike, I might still be waiting on tables, might be an actress, a poet, a comic, a candlestick maker; might have become a crazy cat lady surrounded by overgrown spider plants and empty cartons of fat-free yogurt; might have had a breakdown like my mother, given up like my brother—and Mike might have married Laura New Hampshire (the name we gave the woman who lived across the street from us in New Hampshire who had a major crush on him and would have been a better wife to him because she was more organized and self-sacrificing and in awe of doctors). And I wouldn't be walking around this yard that Mrs. Hart designed with living in mind, wouldn't have those three children inside still counting on me, wouldn't be peering through the plastic-covered windows of the writer's hut thinking, Mausoleum.

Why, when I look at this little, yellow, steep-roofed hut, built for me, am I thinking mausoleum? Is this a sign? Is the fact that Mrs. Hart, the woman I so admired, who inspired me to put down roots, to make a home, died in the bedroom, was wheeled out of the house on a stretcher—Is *that* a sign? Why does everything seem like a sign? I don't know if it's a sign but I *do* know I should object to this extravagant gift, should tell Mike we need to get out of this web of him buying me and me letting him buy me.

I should get a job, a real job, stop wasting my time thinking writing is an actual profession. That any day now I'm going to launch my career. It's a goddamned crapshoot at best. Yes, I *did* want a room of my own. Once. When I still believed that what I had to say would matter to someone other than me. But now it seems a little too late for all that. I need to measure out my time more prudently. Finally figure out what it is I want to do and get it done before the whole goddamned gig is up.

So no, no this isn't how I imagined it. Motherhood is more complex and consuming, but the kids are much more amazing. Quite simply, they taught me how to love. And marriage: There are days when the miracle of what Mike and I have created and endured together astounds me. Days when I am certain, in spite of all our unresolved issues, that this is the man whose body I was meant to bump up against in the middle of the night. But there are days when I know we both feel trapped and the concept of marriage makes no sense to me.

How could one person possibly be lover, friend, roommate, co-parent when the best of each of those roles is intrinsically at odds, and the very things we want and need from one another shift over time? . . . It's too much pressure for me, for him. For anyone.

No, this is not how I imagined it. I'd imagined by forty-five I would have arrived at that Adult Place where you know things and the things you know add up, make sense. Like the inevitable climax in a well-crafted novel (perhaps *that* was the problem with my novel), I was confused about where I was headed—and it didn't add up and instead of a slow climb, it darted all over the goddamned place and felt chaotic and messy and complicated and boring, yes part of it was just god-awful BORING, a never-ending work-in-progress and there probably wasn't enough sex . . . but we stamped all our hands side by side in the wet cement when we patched the driveway, replanted Mrs. Hart's garden beds, made a home that felt like HOME, that reflected all of us, a place where you could put your feet up and eat as much warm apple cake as you wanted and curl into the couch under a worn, crushed-velvet throw and read and laugh or cry.

"You okay?" Mike says, cupping my cold hands in his warm ones, his touch reminding me why I fell in love

with him. His eyes so wide, so open, so willing to absorb all of me, making me feel less cynical, more hopeful, as if with him I can still figure out how to do things
right. He's a good man. I try not to wonder what he saw
in me then, what he could possibly see in me now as we
tuck our hands into my pockets, our fingers instinc-
tively dovetailing into a familiar clasp, and lean against
each other and I nod into his chest and say, "I'm fine
I'm fine I'm fine I'm fine I'm fine," beating time with
my own internal metronome.

thirteen

I'm
My Gramma
Rosie

"**E**VEN THOUGH THE surgeon got clean margins," the oncologist says a few days later, "your risk of invasive cancer is four to five times greater than the average woman."

Mike swallows and bristles at "invasive" and I'm stuck on "average." I've never liked words like "average," such a generic generalization. Who's defining "average," I wonder. Does "average" take into account the list of lifestyle "improvements" I'm making?

"If I exercise more and cut out animal fats and pesticides and decrease my exposure to the electromagnetic field, how does that affect my risk?" I ask the oncologist. I have vowed I will not put one thing in my mouth or on my body that might adversely affect my health. Not counting the drugs and booze from the other night. But from now on. I've done my research and made my own calculations and will re-dedicate myself to clean living and healthy eating.

"Look," the oncologist says, his big droopy lids lowering as he flips the prescription pad upside down and draws several bunches of squiggly circles in a row. "The area was small and noninvasive and we got it all. That's all good." Mike clears his throat, that nervous clearing that tells me he's feeling more anxious about this than I want him to. I want to remind him about the breast cancer chat room where a woman told me I had the "good" cancer.

"Do I need radiation or chemo?" I ask, sweat pooling in the small of my back.

Mike clears his throat several more compulsive times, the oncologist cracks a hairy knuckle on the desk, the fluorescent lights dare me to look at my bare chest.

"No chemo. Radiation is a close call. In fact, I told your husband," he nods at Mike, "that we discussed a case identical to yours in Tumor Board this morning and half the oncologists said they would radiate and half said no. But I think, no." He looks me squarely in the eyes, places a huge, paternal hand over my diminutive one.

Mike holds my other hand as tears well up again. This time from relief.

"These cells," the oncologist says, nodding his head to his drawing, pointing to the first group of squiggly circles labeled *carcinoma in situ,* "are different from these cells." He points to the squiggly circles labeled *invasive cancer.* I'm not sure if it's my middle-aged eyesight or his shoddy drawing skills but they look pretty much the same to me. "They were contained *in* the milk ducts. What we're concerned about is recurrence. Your risk of invasive cancer is 24% over thirty years and the only thing we *do* know *statistically* that will decrease your risk is Tamoxifen. With five years of Tamoxifen you halve your risk."

Tamoxifen. Ah, the dreaded Tamoxifen, the anti-estrogen, a drug designed to trick my body into early menopause, steal away the final years of my younger womanhood, that increases my risk of uterine cancer; cataracts; stroke; pulmonary embolism; not to mention fatigue, bloating, and weight gain; insomnia and mood swings; hot flashes and night sweats. Many websites proclaim its dangers, balk at the hypocrisy of treating cancer risk *with* a cancer risk.

When I was in college, the board game RISK was popular for a while. We'd get stoned and I'd stare at the little plastic pieces moving across the territories and get utterly confused about allies and enemies, arguing that nothing could be that black and white, complicating the whole notion of the game. But I understand that estrogen is my enemy now; the very thing that made me big busted and fertile and a terrific nurser has turned on me, inside my milk ducts where my body incubated nourishment that made my babies pink cheeked and roly-poly thighed. It's all so twisted and ironic and confusing. Tamoxifen, a hero and a hazard, my breasts, a giver and taker of life, and I, the protagonist *and* the antagonist in this story.

"How often do women like me elect to get rid of them?" I ask, ignoring Mike's throat tic, thinking maybe I should just cut my losses. What is the point of hanging on to flesh that might kill me?

"Some women are paralyzed by the diagnosis." He looks at me, glances at my chest. "But I don't see that happening with you. You're handling this fine."

I nod. Try to look "fine" as my mind wanders to waking that morning in disbelief that I had an appointment with an oncologist. Oncologist? That word was for other people, older people, unlucky people. People who die. I stared into my bureau drawers, agonizing over what to wear, wondering why they didn't send *that* information with the postcard appointment reminder and how I was supposed to navigate all these decisions without more guidance? You get an instruction booklet with a toaster oven but no instructions for marriage or motherhood or cancer.

Cancer especially.

Growing up, people didn't talk about it. The word it-self was taboo, as if saying it provoked it. So how was I to know how to *live* it? I thought maybe I should wear Mike's old Dartmouth sweatshirt that he gave me to wear home from his apartment the first time we slept together. We'd been up all night in that I-don't-want-to-close-my-eyes-and-miss-a-second-of-you state of mind and just as I drifted off, he'd tiptoed out to the little patisserie at the corner of 10th and Hudson to buy croissants and cappuccinos. I awoke to him feeding me pieces of warm buttery dough from his fingers. Then he gave me his sweatshirt and I slipped it over my head and smelled Mike, a combination of Ivory soap and Old Spice with just the tiniest hint of beer. And it was big enough to render me shapeless. Amorphous. Possibly not even human. A great big one-celled organism meant to mutate, must mutate to stay alive . . .

"Tamoxifen is the only thing we can offer younger, pre-menopausal women," the oncologist slices into my mind spinning out of control. . . . "It isn't a perfect drug but it's all we have now." He sort of smiles, the corners of his eyes etched with concern. A smile that says he's sorry he has to tell me this.

I glance at the black turtleneck draped across my lap that I wore instead of the sweatshirt and calculate that half of 24% over thirty years still leaves 12%. Think, 12% is pretty high, higher than the odds of getting my novels published. All these years I'd played the low odds in my favor, telling myself that less than 10% was still pretty good odds, convinced I would be in that pool. And now? "Who's to say I won't be in that 12%?" I ask.

He says nothing for a moment and my eyes loop through his name and his M.D. embroidered in cursive over the pocket of his crisp white coat.

"We'll keep a close eye on you," he says. "Back here in three months. Six-month mammograms and check-ups for a few years. You're married to a radiologist so I'm sure we'll get plenty of films." He looks at Mike, who nods and clears his throat again.

I can tell that "We'll keep a close eye on you" is supposed to make me feel better. But it makes me feel like a criminal. A bad girl who needs to be watched. Makes me want to slide off my seat, slip under the door, sneak as far away from me and my cells as I can. I should be relieved. I'm fine. I'm fine. I'm lucky. Luckier than so many others. It could have been so much worse. I'm lucky. I'm lucky. I'm lucky. . . . But I'm worried. I want better odds. I *should* be okay but I might not be.

I glance down and for the first time since the surgery I really look at my breast and am startled by the ragged scars, the swollen flesh, the bloody scabs. I don't recognize this breast; this skin that harbored tainted cells, this me. I want to protest. I want to tell the oncologist it isn't fair. I want to ask him why I don't get credit for all my good cells. I mean, if you think about it, with all those millions of cells it's pretty amazing more bad shit doesn't happen.

I know. I have to stop worrying, get on with life, pull myself together. One foot in front of the other. I know how to do that. I did that after my parents' divorce, my mother's breakdown, my brother's suicide, but could someone, anyone explain how I am supposed to live in three- and six-month increments without losing my mind, without letting the threat of one stray mutant cell destroy my spirit?

He flips his pad back over and scribbles *Tamoxifen.* "Once a day," he says.

And I realize this is what he has to offer.

"I could walk out of here and be run over by a car in the parking lot," I say as he tears the prescription from the sticky bind and hands it to me.

He nods and pats my hand again, his big dark eyes finally softening, as if this were the very thing he was meaning to say all along.

"This is good, right?" I say to Mike and press the down button and we wait for the numbers to rise.

"Right," Mike says.

"You mean it?" I say inside the elevator as we descend.

"Sure."

"Really?"

"Uh-huh."

"Then why do you have that look on your face? Why do you keep clearing your throat?"

He clears his throat and says, "Allergies?"

The doors open and I grasp his hand and say, "I mean do you really really really mean it?"

"What do you want?" he says, stepping out of the elevator and leading us past the framed watercolors of something soft hued, around the circular information desk, into the vestibule piled high with free periodicals: *The Isthmus, The Onion, Wisconsin Woman, Maximum Ink, Sustainable Times.*

"I want better answers," I say, tucking one of each under my arm. "I want to know why this happened. To *me.*" I point to my chest. "It still doesn't make sense to me and . . . I want to know if you think I should have them taken off before it's too late."

He doesn't say anything as we exit the building and head toward the parking lot where we find our car exactly where we left it, giving me a moment of relief. Our car. It's here. Waiting for us. Just like we expected. Life hasn't veered too far from where it was.

In the car, before Mike puts the key into the ignition, he rolls his palm back and forth on the steering wheel and stares straight ahead. "This is hard for me, too," he finally says.

"What? Talking about removing my breasts?"

He shudders. More rolling, his wedding ring clanking rhythmically.

"Does that mean yes?"

"It means I'm having a hard time believing this is us," he says. "That we're talking about you."

An elderly couple shuffles by and I think about last New Year's Eve day and how that morning I ran past a couple walking through the neighborhood. I thought when we first moved in they were probably just a little older than us and now they looked so much older, it shocked me.

I tried to explain that to Mike that day but he had snapped, "I can't believe you're saying that. As if you're above aging. We're all aging. Ever since my knee surgery, I haven't felt the same. Do you know how that feels? Of course you don't. You *never* get sick. . . . "

I wanted to say more. I wanted to tell him how all day I was tempted to stop people in their seventies and eighties on the street and ask them how they lived knowing each day that this could be the end. Little did I know that I'd be facing the same questions before the month was over. Or *did* my body know? Was that why I leapt from middle-aged musings to eighty-year-olds?

But at that moment, Mike was scowling at me, ending the discussion because it made *him* feel older. Later that night at my friend's party, I joked that this year I was planning to hold steady at forty-five. My friend's sister said maybe we could all back up a few years, and she did the Michael Jackson Moon Dance backwards and then in place—and we all laughed so hard we cried.

"You've always been the healthy one," he says now. "I counted on that, too."

"I'm sorry," I say, feeling just like I did the summer I turned seventeen and was driving to California with a carload of friends when we got into a bad accident on the south side of Chicago. Everyone was okay but my car was totaled; and all I could think was *They were counting on me for a ride* and I couldn't stop apologizing for inconveniencing them.

Although I pretty much got over that after I met Surfer Boy in San Diego a few weeks later. We fell in love-at-first-sight love and spent the rest of the summer in one long riveting conversation that never ended. When I went back East in the fall, he wrote me love letters, quoting poems I'd mentioned briefly—*all* of John Donne's minor sonnets in his vigorously sloppy hand. He wanted me to transfer to San Diego State and I almost did, but then panicked, thinking I was too young to be so "involved." I broke up with him, and he married the following year. Years later, after *I'd* married, Mike found his love letters and was so jealous that he burned them. And I didn't stop him.

"A mastectomy is major surgery," Mike says now. "And there's always risk and possible complications with that . . . lymphedema, for one thing, causing permanent swelling and limited range of motion in your arms and then sometimes they find cancer in the chest wall. . . . "

Chest wall? I hadn't visualized flesh being cut away to a wall. The bone. My shoulders buckle at the image.

"So even then there is a slight chance," he continues, reminding me a mastectomy doesn't eliminate my risk entirely, that no matter how I try to spin this, it always lands on uncertainty.

"I just want to know what else I can do. If I'm doing all the right things. If I'm taking more of a risk *with* the Tamoxifen, if. . . . "

"I don't know," he says, "I wish I had the answers."

"I know *you* don't know. I'm not asking you as a doctor. I'm trying to talk to you about this as my husband."

"That's the tricky thing with cancer, we just don't know. We know your risks. Your options."

"It isn't enough," I say. "I want more. . . . "

We both stare out the window, the keys perched on the seat between us.

"I don't want you to get mad about this," I say. "And it isn't that I have anything against Lakeview or your colleagues but . . . I'd like to go for a second opinion to one of those really big cancer places. Sloan Kettering or M.D. Anderson. Just to make sure I'm doing everything."

I watch the elderly couple, elbows locked, still making their way across the parking lot, as if they have all the time in the world, as if where they are going is no more or less important than where they are.

"How about Mayo?" he asks.

"Really?"

He nods. "Sure. Why not? I'm pretty sure Bruce Weiner's son works there. I'll call him and set something up."

"Really?" I say. And before he can answer, "Really?" Again.

He nods, clanks his ring a few more times on the wheel before picking up the keys.

"That would be great," I say as we back out of the parking space.

I measure my life in Tamoxifen tabs. I shake the little white pill into my palm, after my cup of warm water with lemon (which Deepak Chopra recommends first thing in the morning to cleanse and detoxify) and organic fresh fruit, but before my whole-grain steel-cut oats, and think, I'm my Gramma Rosie.

The one who took so many prescription medications that she bought a diamond-encrusted pill box in their honor. The one who was widowed in her early fifties after my grandfather died of lung cancer, who lived alone in a fancy high-rise with wall-to-wall gold carpet and tightly upholstered white-on-white furniture and silk lampshades covered in plastic and a kidney-shaped, built-in swimming pool (which I dove into once and smashed my braces into my lips), who taught me a mean game of gin rummy and how to make Boston Cream Pie from a box, who died young but always looked old, who wore a girdle and kept her false teeth in a Waterford crystal highball glass by her bedside table, who paid us to visit her because she was so lonely.

Who, I thought, until recently, had all those medical problems because she ate crap and didn't exercise and chain-smoked extra-long mentholated Virginia Slims, while my son bragged to his friends, "My mother can run up all the hills in the neighborhood." I pop the Tamoxifen in my mouth; try not to think about my risk of stroking out. I'm my Gramma Rosie and there's nothing I can do about it.

"You are *not* Rose Applebaum," my mother shouts into the phone when I share this insight with her.

She calls several times a week now. When I answer the phone, she always says, "You okay, honey?" As if I'm an invalid. My mother, who is overweight and a smoker and hasn't exercised since 1989 and used to call me with all her hypochondriacal concerns, now keeps telling me how healthy she is for nearly seventy. I think it's supposed to make me feel better (about my genes?) but it actually makes me feel worse, like my body must really be fucked up if it can't stay healthy with all my concentrated effort.

Last week, when I told her I was going to Mayo for a second opinion, she said, "Thank the Lord." We're Jewish, but my mother is highly "experimental" with religion. She's been a Buddhist, a Born Again, an Evangelical and now she's talking about converting to Catholicism (something about the intellectual depth of mysticism). And she has a very old-fashioned view of doctors. She thinks great doctors are Gods, that they have the means and the power to reverse your fate, which was why she was so thrilled I was going to Mayo. "They'll take *care* of you," she said.

I'm not saying *I* believed that.

But I'm not saying I didn't entirely, either.

"Did I ever tell you about when your father and I lived with your grandmother Rosie?" she says now, "and she removed all the doors in the house? *That's* the craziness from your father's side of the family. You wouldn't do that. You need to stop thinking negative thoughts. You need to work on purging your negativity. Talk to your Mayo people about that. . . . "

fourteen

Family Vacation

A FEW WEEKS later, in March, we're on our way to Laguna Beach for our family vacation. Anna chose the destination back in December when we'd envisioned this break as recovery from the college application ordeal. We all wanted something mindless and beachy and there was the added possibility of movie star sightings. According to the girls, Steven on *Laguna Beach* is *very* hot—although Mike claims he isn't technically a movie star since it's a reality show and he also thinks chasing celebrities is "a foolish waste of time."

He's probably right, but we're planning a day in L.A. to shop and stalk anyway. We've booked two adjoining rooms at the Ritz Carlton with ocean views on the club level, and upgraded to Business Class, all of which makes me suspicious of how sure Mike is that I'm going to be okay. All this extravagance and he's back to being so damn nice to me all the time, even when I can tell I'm annoying the hell out of him.

As the plane picks up speed down the runway, Mike reaches for *SkyMall* and I pop another organic fruit juice and brown rice syrup sweetened throat lozenge into my mouth and think about the Midwest Dance Competition in Chicago I took Maddy to last January, the week before my mammogram. We decided to take the bus with the rest of the dance team because it seemed like the friendly, team-like thing to do. But when the mom with the full-length fur coat and collagen-bitten lips sauntered onto the bus and I glanced over at the woman taking the seat next to me and the one across the aisle and noticed they'd all had their hair professionally done and were wearing expensive pressed slacks and polished loafers (while I had worn my running clothes and baseball cap thinking I could get a quick run in before the "team" dinner), I realized not only was I dressed all wrong but I was way out of my league.

I buried my head in my book, but the smell of formaldehyde distracted me, burning my eyes and nostrils. I turned to Maddy seated between two dancers painting their toenails and we locked eyes and she mouthed, "Can you believe this?"

The hotel lobby was crawling with dyed-blond girls in skimpy sequined costumes bossing around plump mothers who stuffed French fries in their mouths with one hand and sprayed their daughters' dos with the other. This was not about dance. This was a beauty pageant with shimmies. A world that made me wonder if there actually *had* been a women's movement thirty years earlier.

"Furs and formaldehyde" is what I say to Mike now as the wheels tuck into the plane.

He looks up from *SkyMall,* which he is studying as if it's a medical textbook.

"I will never use nail polish again. Do you know how carcinogenic formaldehyde is?" This is just one of many interesting pieces of information that I've learned while Googling recently. My fascination with the effect of chemicals on cellular integrity means I either missed my calling as a chemist or I'm pathologically obsessed with my cells.

He nods, pressing his index finger on a turquoise motorized pool lounger.

In Business Class the booze is free-flowing (even though it's not even 11 A.M.). A boisterous couple behind us are on their second glass of champagne and the woman is laughing so heartily, for a moment I think I should just get smashed and be more like her. I should be like George on that *Seinfeld* episode when he decided to do the opposite of everything he thought he should do.

"Do you think they have any bottled water in glass containers?" I ask Mike instead.

"I doubt it," he says, dog-earing the *SkyMall* page.

The flight attendant overhears me and shakes her head, looking disappointed that I'm not inquiring about a "real" drink and asks the other couple if they'd like a refill.

"Of course!" they say. More toasting. More cheers. "To refills."

"Those clouds look like cauliflower," the woman says and laughs, and I think, Cauliflower is one of the cruciferous vegetables I should eat daily to decrease my risk. Cauliflower, broccoli, brussels sprouts, cabbage . . . I wonder if Mike wishes I were more like her and why isn't this sore throat going away?

"Plastic from water bottles can leach into the water molecules and plastics act like a xenoestrogen in the body," I say to Mike.

"Xenoestrogen? What the hell is that?"

"It's the 'bad' kind of estrogen, the kind that can cause breast cancer, the kind that is like poison to me. How do you not know that? Didn't they teach you anything in medical school?"

I'm waiting for him to lose patience with me. Instead he nods and pats my hand and says, "You're going to be okay. . . . What do you think of this?" He points to the motorized raft.

When the lunch menus arrive, the couple ohh and ahh over the choices, halibut in a light garlic sauce with roasted red pepper polenta or grilled chicken with shitake mushrooms and jasmine rice. I shake my head—microwaved and filled with trans fats, pesticides, and hormones? I don't think so.

"To plane food," the woman says, clinking another glass.

Mike tells the flight attendant he'll take *both* our meals *and* a Heineken *and* a glass of red wine. She seems a little happier with us until she sees me pass out bags of raw nuts and seeds and raisins to the children who are in a row across the aisle listening to their iPods and reading. They order their own meals and stuff the bags in their seat pockets.

"Could we buy some avocados?" I ask as soon as we land in L.A.

"The radiation from the plane," I say to Mike's puzzled face, as if *he's* the crazy one. "I read you can offset some of the radiation by eating avocados—of course they have to be organic."

●   ●   ●

A few days before we left, a month post-surgery, I was given the go-ahead by my surgeon to run again. So in

Laguna that's what I do. I run (thirty minutes or more of exercise a day is associated with a lower rate of recurrence) and go to exercise classes at the hotel's fitness center with the girls and walk the beach with Alex, tossing a ball, anything to keep moving so I don't feel so awful that I'm not enjoying this last family vacation with Anna.

When we planned this trip, I'd pictured us all relaxing and romping and sipping cool, fruity drinks under cabanas. But it's in the low sixties and we sit by the ocean, wrapped in towels, cupping warm tea, the kids arguing over who kicked sand in whose face and when Mike asks me if I want to go on an all-day deep-sea fishing trip (even though he knows I hate fishing), I remind myself that family vacations are often most enjoyable in the glossy brochure stage.

Last time we went on vacation was to Palm Beach more than a year ago. It was June, off season, so the flight and the hotel were a bargain, although it was unbearably hot and the hotel was hosting a convention of women from Dallas who sold fruit- and flower-print-inspired clothing out of their homes at Tupperware-type parties. They monopolized the lobby, debating marketing strategies in cherry-printed shifts and daisy-splattered skirts with matching earrings and strappy high-heeled sandals, their hair and nails perfectly coiffed.

I'd wanted to go to Palm Beach because my friend Allison (my best friend in NYC) lived a few towns over and I hadn't seen her in more than ten years. Coincidentally, my younger brother was at a Club Med nearby for *his* family vacation. He'd been friends with Allison, having met her at my apartment years ago and had stayed in touch with her ex-husband over business. So he drove up to Palm Beach for the night and we all arranged to meet at her ex's restaurant. It seemed a little odd that we were meeting at her ex's place, but Allison admitted it was the best restaurant in the area and said she didn't mind. In fact, she said, she could drop her kids with him for visitation and grab a bite to eat with us. Allison was the friend who knew Mike *before* I did. They were both working at the restaurant I had worked at also and would soon work at again (after the Yeshiva where I was teaching stopped paying me because the head Rabbi was absconding the funds).

But at that time, *they* were working together and she invited me to a birthday party for the head dishwasher—one of the many lecherous but ultimately harmless kitchen staff—and he spent the night trying to rub up against my arm while I swatted him away and Mike so chivalrously warned him to back off that I thought maybe he was mocking chivalry. But in the bathroom Allison said she could tell Mike wanted me and even though I wasn't sure I wanted him (or anyone for that matter, I was going through an I'm-sick-of-dating phase) and thought maybe there was something between *them,* once I started working with him, *we* fell in love. Later, when Allison married that schmuck who left her for the manicurist, I wondered if *she* should have ended up with Mike.

"How are you?" Mitch, her ex, the schmuck, said to me that night as he greeted us at our table with the most elaborate tray of appetizers I'd ever seen.

"Great," I said. "How are you?"

"Same old same old," he said, looking the same. He hadn't aged at all, the little-boy face still little-boyish, other than a slightly receding hairline. I wanted to tell him he was a son-of-a-bitch asshole for fucking around on my friend, but I spotted Allison out the front window, in the parking lot, and felt strange and guilty for talking to him—for being in the restaurant, period.

My brother walked up then and slapped Mitch on the back and I walked to the door to greet her.

"I'm coming from work," she said, nodding to her off-white linen suit. She'd started selling real estate after her marriage fell apart and I was struck by how professional she looked. Her hair neatly blown dry, her shoes and bag matching, her eyes delicately shadowed.

"You look great," I said, feeling self-conscious about my tight, low-rise jeans and tank top and wind-blown do. She was a grown-up now and I . . . what was I?

And then we were all drinking and laughing and the food didn't stop; oyster shots and duck and mango sushi rolled in caviar and raw tuna and avocado salad and platters of delicately grilled fish and fresh pasta, and my girls loved her. I could see that they could see me in her and her in me, certain phrases and expressions that we'd rubbed into one another, the way best friends do.

And I also could see how much she and Mike enjoyed each other and I wondered how much of the her in me is what he'd been attracted to. I was thinking that she was thinking that I'd made the better choice and that made all the difference and I wondered, Was I to blame for her misfortune? Could I have prevented it? By giving her Mike? Could I give her Mike now?

*   *   *

In Laguna, we meet a couple at breakfast. The woman, a flamboyant makeup artist from Oklahoma, is telling us a story about doing makeup for some famous sports figure. "You wouldn't think he needed a makeup person, but he did. Big time!" And then she's telling us about her first husband, whom she married at sixteen because the condom broke but that she was smart enough to leave by seventeen, and now she has a grown son.

"Believe it or not!" She sucks in her highlighted cheeks and gushes about how she met her current husband— the one polishing off another mimosa and alternately reading the editorial page of the newspaper and smiling at her affectionately—who was the best thing that ever happened to her and now she (or they, she *should* say, she says) are trying, desperately, to get pregnant.

"I tried standing on my head after our last 'session,'" she says, using her fingers to air quote "session." "But I landed on my back. . . . " When she pauses to take a breath, I feel this pressure to "share," too. Tell her that I've recently had breast surgery and I have a lingering cold and an outrageous fear of recurrence, which is making me think that if I keep sitting here I will miss my 9 A.M. Pilates—and who knows what kind of irrevocable havoc that will wreak on my cells—and that I used to be more fun or at least I think I was before I became so goddamned literal. But now I'm convinced that every single thing I do or don't do, every piece of food that crosses my lips, every substance that touches my skin will either hurt or heal me. But I don't "share" because I realize I don't want her or anyone to know I've had cancer, just thinking about that word makes me feel like a leper. In fact, I'm so sure if I let her see me even one second longer she will know, whether or not I tell, that I excuse myself and run and cry all the way to the fitness center.

Later that morning, Mike suggests I skip my afternoon exercise and we go out with the couple we met at breakfast for Mexican and margaritas instead. I blow up at him; accuse him of not wanting me to get healthy.

At The Ivy in Santa Monica (where we've come to find the stars after a day of shopping on Melrose Place and poking around Beverly Hills where we didn't spot anyone except half a dozen girls who *looked* like Jessica Simpson), Maddy thinks she sees Meg Ryan heading into the bathroom.

"Did you see her?" she asks me.

I shake my head.

"I think it's her, but I'm not sure. . . . Go in the bathroom and see."

"I just went to the bathroom," I say.

"Come on. You have to," she says, nudging me.

I get up and walk across the restaurant and when I open the door to the tiny bathroom, there is a woman, tall and very slim, even though she's wrapped in lots of loopy layers and an enormous head of hair, waiting her turn. She glances toward me, but barely, and I recognize the famous lip pout. It *is* her. It's Meg Ryan and I'm starstruck.

What to say? What to say? "I ADORE you," I blurt out. She averts her eyes, turns her head, and flips her long, wavy mane of hair all over the goddamned place, completely ignoring me. As soon as she heads into the stall, I race out of the bathroom, pushing past patrons and wait staff, yelling, "It's her! It's her! Go. Go now! She's peeing!" I shove the girls out of their seats.

They go and are, of course, much cooler than I am, pretending they don't know who she is, getting a good long look at her in the shared mirror over the sink.

"She's had surgery," Anna says, trying to make me feel better.

"I don't really adore her," I say. "I mean, I think she was cute in *When Harry Met Sally* and *Sleepless in Seattle* but that isn't exactly adore."

"I ADORE you," Alex says and I do several more renditions of the hair flip and we can't stop laughing. It's the first time I've laughed really hard since my surgery even though we're laughing at me, the Midwestern Woman Stalking the Celebrity, I'm relieved I remember how.

On the way home, in Minneapolis, where we're changing planes, Mike and the kids go off to buy coffee and munchies and I stay with our bags at the gate. I am just about to put my iPod headphones on when a friend and neighbor from Madison, Dawn Myers, approaches me. I've only recently gotten to know her since she joined our couples book group. But I've known *of* her for years.

She's a brilliant scientist, who has already been awarded more prestigious prizes and honors than anyone I know. She's been married and divorced more than once (which I think takes an enormous amount of courage and faith in love) and she has a boyfriend. Just the word "boyfriend" sounds so exciting. Athletic and slim, she has degrees from a few different Ivy League schools and either Oxford or Cambridge and lived in Europe. She's very up on books and movies and politics (an ardent Bush hater and equally ardent atheist), and she's full of energy, always jetting off somewhere. Skiing and sailing and being flown all over the world to give lectures.

But she's also fun and funny. She couldn't stop giggling as she told me that the last time she flew out East, she was reading *The End of Faith,* the man on the end was reading *The Bible,* and her son was reading *Religion for Dummies.* But the thing I most admire about her is her drive, her ability to see what she wants, career- or love-wise, and to go for it, no dicking around. At the airport she walks up to me with a concerned look on her face. She's heard about my surgery and how *am* I? I tell her other than this lingering cold, I'm fine.

"Well, *that's* a relief," she says again and again as she walks with the gait of a slim twelve-year-old back to her bags and laptop.

I put my headphones on and click on "Stairway to Heaven," and look up to see Mike and the kids walking toward me. They're all laughing about something; they look more relaxed and happier. The kids seem older and I see me in Anna, something around the mouth and eyes. Mike seems surer of his role as father. And then molecules and atoms shift, the world flips upside down and inside out and I realize I'm seeing the future.

Them without me.

I stand up, rip the earplugs out and run to them, abandoning our bags, nearly tripping over my feet.

"What's wrong?" Mike asks.

I'm crying. Hard. Choking on fear.

"Nothing," I say, wedging myself in the middle. "I just missed you guys."

fifteen

Of Yogis and Sages, Semantics and Guarantees

M Y BROTHER DANIEL'S high school girlfriend Jenny was one of those pretty, popular girls, with hair like a lioness and commanding green eyes and a ravenous smile, a girl who was always throwing her arms around people, like Daniel, making him think that her touch guaranteed his happiness.

And a month after he went off to college, she screwed around on him with this All-City basketball player. I knew she was screwing around because I saw her at parties consuming the other guy, but I never told my brother because . . . I was trying to protect him? I was a coward? Indifferent? I'm not sure.

But, he found out soon enough, and it broke his heart and his spirit. Two years later he was ranting through the streets of L.A. claiming to be Jesus, and my dad had to wrestle him home in a straightjacket. Now I wonder, at 4:37 A.M., if the Jenny thing could have been what tipped him over the edge. I run scenarios through my head: *If Daniel hadn't found out. If she'd never met the basketball guy. If Daniel'd never met her. If she'd never been born.* I flip them back and forth and inside and out and then at some point, after what feels like hours, I fall into a heavy black sleep—and wake to Mike's empty, rumpled side of the bed and the groans and clank of the house already in gear.

Downstairs the children huddle around the island munching buttered toast and bowls of granola. They barely look up as I slip into the kitchen and think, They're more independent than they were the first time I had a breast scare in 2001, when all I could think was that there was no way they could survive without me. Not only were they all much younger, Alex only five, but they were more attached emotionally and physically to me. Mike was so busy making his way in the new practice and had worked such long hours through most of their childhoods, the girls still treated him a bit suspiciously. And while Alex clearly adored him, they hadn't bonded over the Red Sox and ESPN or begun their nonstop Little League dialogue in secret code: "Make him a hitter." "Keep it in the strike zone." "He took one for the team."

But I was also a different kind of mother back then because I was so worried about my ability to mother, I overperformed, thought it my job to fix life for them; to make friends friendlier and teachers more compelling and appreciative; to convince the entire world to love and protect them; to soften all the sharp edges, so they wouldn't have to feel pain. Until I realized I couldn't. Shouldn't. Although that realization ebbs and flows.

Just a couple of months ago, at the Midwest Dance Competition, when Maddy took off her jazz shoes, the sight of her bunions and bruises sent a sharp pang through me, as if her feet were mine. How had I allowed her lovely little unblemished baby toes to reach this state of neglect? Until I remembered that the best dancers have the ugliest feet. And that she wasn't a baby. And her toes were her own.

But now as they read the paper and clear and load their dishes and start the morning search for notebooks and shin pads and lunch bags, no one asking me where, no one complaining about another day at school that I know they all have complaints about, I wonder if a slow fade away isn't kinder so by the time I am gone (*whenever* that is) it won't be such a shock.

I kiss and wave them off to school from the front door, muttering, "Did you brush your teeth?" as their backpacks and messenger bags bounce down the driveway. Then climb the stairs to get dressed for the day.

I put on my running shorts and tank, my Black Dog baseball cap, my Survival of the Fittest running socks (that used to amuse me but now make me wonder if I'm qualified to wear them) and tie my shoes. I meet Martha—my cooler, triathlete friend, the one who wants me to run the NYC Half-Marathon with her in August—at the trail and plod behind her, happy to listen to a story about one of the college-aged guys she works with at Movin' Shoes and his girlfriend woes. Something about how they were "friends with benefits," but now he wants something more and she doesn't. I think it involves him crying. Or is it lying? I'm concentrating so hard on my breathing I'm not hearing everything.

She races even farther ahead of me. I hunker down to keep up.

"How about the half-marathon?" she says. "You in?"

"I don't know." I try to hide my panting. But the pace is too strenuous. I'm not back in shape. I still tire easily and am nursing this cold and wondering why it's hanging on. But I don't say this. I don't want to sound like a wimp, so instead I say, "Maybe I'll start training and see how that goes."

After the run I stand at my back door and stare at the hut and clutch the moleskin journal Mike bought me in my still sweaty hands, and think, I should go out to the hut and write. I should write. I should.

I should either revise the new novel or the old novel or start another novel. Or a story. A short story. A poem. Haiku? One line. A word. But I don't.

I have no word.

Nothing to say.

I mosey back into the house and sink into the soft salmon-colored chair by the large window in the family room and count knots in the split-rail fence. I fiddle with my notebook, open and close and open it and count how many lines are on the page. Click my pen on and off and on and off and on. Roll the inky round ball over the page, feel the metal tip vibrate through my finger tips and my hand shake as details of the scare pour out until I'm trembling and weeping and curling into a fetal ball and falling asleep . . . and wake stung raw.

Papers from Mayo arrive in thick white envelopes that are oddly about the same size and weight as short stories returned for rejection. Only instead of "While there is much to be admired, this isn't quite right for us" letters, these are stuffed with forms to fill out. Instructions about chest x-rays and fasting blood tests and reminders to keep the few days after the appointment free "just in case" I need further testing, hospitalization. Questions about religious preferences and living wills. Living wills?

I'm thinking they've made a mistake. They're treating me as if I'm sicker than I am. I call the *if you have any further questions regarding your appointment* number to explain: "They got it all out. I'm just coming for a consultation to make sure we're doing everything possible to prevent. . . . "

"This is procedural," the overly officious voice on the other end says. "Everyone is treated the same." No inflection. "Can we count on you for research if you qualify?"

"Sure," I say, afraid to cross this woman. Convinced she holds my fate in her pen-wielding hand.

I hang up the phone and stare at the living-will space and think of my friend Allison's sister who threw herself out a window, after their mother died of cancer, and ended up in a coma. Allison dutifully visited her sister every day, put her own life into a kind of coma, spending most of her free time at the hospital racked with guilt about her sister's fate and her inability to do anything about it other than visit. I went with her once, but as soon as we got to the hospital room door and I caught a glimpse inside—the tubes, the steady beat and erratic flash of the breathing machine, the rubbery cheeks—I couldn't step over the threshold.

Now, I stare at the box on the form and think I should relay *this* story on *this* form but there isn't any room for explanations, no space other than a small box to check. *Do you have a living will?* Yes or no. Me, a living will? My parents haven't even been seriously sick yet. Why do I keep feeling shocked that I have to worry about my health? Why can't I adjust? Figure out how to read these forms and fill in the goddamned blanks without falling apart?

I shove the papers aside and inch my way over to the computer to add to my list of *Keys To NOT Being That 12%* that I plan to bring to my Mayo visit, to show them how dedicated I am to Living.

1. Eat only organic (even if this means I can't eat out or travel or leave the house if I'm hungry). Small price to pay for life!
2. Avoid animal fats or proteins (there is a theory that animal fat and possibly protein is one of the main culprits behind cancer). So no meat, no butter, no cheese, no ice cream. No ice cream? No ice cream.
3. Avoid sugar (some sites claim sugar feeds cancer— something to do with fermentation?). Maybe all sugar except a little chocolate. Chocolate has antioxidants.
4. Eat more Super Foods. According to Steven Pratt, there are fourteen Super Foods: beans, blueberries, broccoli, oats, oranges, pumpkin, salmon, soy, spinach, tea, tomatoes, turkey, walnuts, and yogurt. I cross out soy (because I was told by my first breast surgeon in 2001 to avoid it since some studies show soy might increase the risk of breast cancer) and turkey and yogurt (because I'm avoiding animal protein), which leaves me with eleven foods. Maybe *only* eat these eleven foods. Who needs other foods? Are other foods necessary? Look this up.
5. Except flax. Flax is in its own category of Super Food (not on Steven Pratt's list but on many other lists). Flax is the Superest of Super Foods. Continue to sprinkle flax on *everything*.
6. Exercise more. If 30–60 minutes of exercise decreases my risk, wouldn't it make sense that 60–90 minutes would

double that decrease? Every time I think about ice cream, exercise instead.

7. Meditate. I read that people who meditate have a lower rate of recurrence (although when I try to meditate it makes my mind race faster, makes me want to check e-mail and think about all the phone calls I have to make and errands I need to run). Work on that.

8. Do more yoga because I read that people who do yoga also have a lower recurrence rate although I'm not sure if that means people who do yoga and meditate as separate activities or who meditate while they do yoga. I wonder if it counts that I do yoga mostly for the workout. I mean, I get the mind/body stuff but mostly I want to sweat and stay flexible and by the time we get to shavasana at the end of class, I'm already making lists in my head. What's up with all the lists in my head? Are lists linked to rate of recurrence? Check this.

9. Live a more purposeful life. I read that people who have a sense of purpose live longer. Purpose? Purpose? I thought my purpose was to write but now I'm not so sure. In fact, writing has often made me feel *not* purposeful; the end product has such an uncertain life. After all, what is the worth of words and ideas stuffed in bins under my desk other than a waste of paper and space and time? Does a thought even exist if there is no one on the other side to receive it? Maybe I should do something with my hands. I always thought carpenters must feel purposeful. They make something useful. Maybe I should take up carpentry. Look into carpentry.

I glance at my list, feeling more confident and in control. Screw those Mayo forms. Screw that 12%. That 12% isn't going to get me. I can use this list to make absolutely sure I'm NOT that 12%. I stare at the screen and click on a site that says PLANT ESTROGENS and find this: *Plant estrogens act like natural estrogen in the body and while some studies indicate they may decrease the risk of breast cancer others indicate they may in fact increase the risk of breast cancer (especially soy).* Okay, I knew about soy. But the list of plant estrogens includes most fruits and legumes and green vegetables (especially all the cruciferous vegetables—the ones I have been overloading on because I'd read they flush estrogen from the body) as well as whole grains, nuts, and seeds (especially flax). Flax? I scroll down and find BORONS. Borons? Borons, which include all green vegetables, fruit, nuts, pears, apples, raisins, and tomatoes, also have estrogen-like properties.

My heart is racing, my mind flipping, my stomach gurgling. Most of the foods I thought were healthy may be harmful; well, they could be helpful but only in certain amounts although no one knows the exact amounts.

What the hell am I supposed to eat? How do I know what to place between my lips and swallow? How did one of life's pleasures morph into this complicated, possibly deadly pursuit? I love food and eating. I grew up in a family dedicated to meals; halfway through breakfast we were already discussing the possibilities for lunch and dinner.

My mother and I could analyze the intricacies of a perfect pear with the same zeal that we discussed Sartre and there is a chunky apple walnut cake with a warm apple cider brown sugar Calvados glaze that I always make in the fall after we go apple picking that I have literally dreamt about. But apples and walnuts are plant estrogens *and* borons, and butter and sugar. . . . I stare at my list of SUPER FOODS and cross-reference it with the list of plant estrogens and borons.

I end up with two things I'm pretty sure I can safely ingest: filtered water and organic green tea.

The drive to the Mayo Clinic in Rochester, Minnesota is 240 miles.

Mike and I leave at 4 A.M. in pitch black and drive in silence past corn and soy fields and sheaves of hay, over dark swaths of tarred road so long and straight it's hard to tell how far we've come, how far we still need to go, until we reach the Mississippi where the land softens and begins to undulate in the early-morning April light.

The night before we left for Mayo, I laid in bed wide awake, counting the seconds between Mike's snores as if they were labor contractions and thinking about what I would eat for breakfast if I weren't paranoid about eating and didn't have to fast because I was having my blood tested for every possible value in the morning: I'd have one of Mike's omelettes (he is the *best* after-sex omelette maker) with freshly squeezed orange juice and those real English Muffins dotted with little pockets begging to be filled with butter and jam. Of course there would have to be a little bit of chocolate at the end, maybe just a truffle or two.

Rochester, Minnesota is a nondescript town, marked by strip malls and fast food franchises and signs to the

Mayo Clinic and St. Mary's Hospital. Once you hit downtown it's obvious that Rochester is all about Mayo: buildings and walkways and white-coated health professionals and patients in wheelchairs and walkers, the entire town looking like it could be a movie set for a new doctor show. A show about people, ordinary people, who come here to be tested for stuff they can't study for.

We park and follow the signs to the Gondola building to check in and as we head down the wide marble and glass hallways lined in original Andy Warhol silk-screened flower prints and clusters of earnest-looking doctors and nurses discussing cases in hushed tones, the weight and the prominence of Mayo swaddles me, makes me think maybe my mother is right, maybe this place is the Home of Gods. Mike stops at the plaque of donors and I see a wistful look in his eye as he reads it.

"What are you thinking?" I ask him.

"You don't want to hear this. . . . " he says.

"No, I do. Tell me."

"It's nothing," he says. "Let's go find hematology."

"No. Tell me," I say.

"There's just something so substantial feeling here," he says, pointing to the plaque. "Something I miss being a part of."

I nod and think about how I chided Mike for the sense of security and superiority Dartmouth and his fraternity and secret society gave him. "The people at Dartmouth are no smarter or better than the people at the University of Toledo," I always said. "The power of an institution is upheld and perpetuated by those who have a vested interest in maintaining the power." But now, now I want to believe that an institution, like Mayo, really is superior enough to protect me.

I submit to the blood test. What choice do I have? That's the thing about being a patient: You're forced into such a passive role and there's really nothing you can do but follow the phlebotomist to the chair, state your name and birth date, rest your elbow on the tray table, let her dab antiseptic wipe on your arm and squeeze it with a rubber band until your vein pops.

I let them shoo me to radiology where they have me strip to a cotton gown and stand against an x-ray film, breathe in and hold as they take a picture of my chest. Should I smile? Is this more like a mug shot or a passport photo? Will they be able to tell I smoked in college and does that explain the cold, the cough that's still lingering?

A few hours later, while waiting in the office in a stiff patient chair, I'm bracing myself for the news that they've found cancer in my lungs and that my blood reveals problems I can't even begin to comprehend.

But the oncologist says that their pathologists reread all my slides and read my recent pathology as atypical ductal hyperplasia. "But they upgraded your benign 2001 diagnosis to atypical lobular hyperplasia. And your 2003 core showed proliferative changes," she says.

I'm a little confused. Is this good news? Can I throw my Gramma Rosie pills away? "Meaning?" I say.

"It's a spectrum, subjective, a matter of a cell or two difference and you have quite a medical history: seven biopsies in five years, two cases of cellular mutation and your breasts are dense and your young age. . . . " She looks at the computer screen and squints a moment before she says, "In fact, your risk of invasive cancer is slightly higher than your Lakeview oncologist told you." She points to the computer screen and I glance at the chart and numbers but don't really "see" them. "We recommend you stay on the Tamoxifen and close monitoring and return in three months for your six-month post-surgical mammogram."

"Okay," I say and nod. What else can I do? I can't argue. She's the expert. But I pull my Healthy Living List from my bag. "I have a few more questions," I say. "I'm wondering what else I can do. I thought I was doing everything to stay healthy but obviously I missed something. So I've been researching. . . . "

We both stare down at my four pages of notes and the oncologist says, "Would you like to see the nutritionist?"

The whole way down the hall, Mike's tension is palpable. "Mayo's interpretation of your slides is a matter of semantics," he finally says.

"Semantics? I love semantics. I live for semantics."

"Do you understand? It's a spectrum. A difference of a cell or two."

"Is it Mayo?" I ask him. "Are you upset with Mayo because Mayo makes you feel worse about practicing medicine in Madison?"

He looks stunned for a moment and I wish I hadn't thrown that back in his face. But I'm not feeling big enough to take it back.

"No, No, No, . . . " he says. "George [the Lakeview pathologist who read my slides] is the best pathologist in Madison. He's as good as anyone at Mayo. I trust his judgment and he sent it out to a national expert and they *both* called it intermediate-grade DCIS. That is not something to mess around with, which is why I wanted to get it out fast and I wanted wide, clean margins. Just last week, I read a film of a woman less severe than you, one case of atypical hyperplasia and at her follow-up they found invasive cancer. Already metastasized into the liver. Cancer is a mystery. The only difference any of this makes is that we might have treated your 2001 scare more aggressively and 28%? Did you hear what she said? Your risk, according to Mayo, is *higher* than we thought. . . . "

I didn't hear that. Can't wrap my brain around 28%. That's getting up there. Well, halved to 14% with the drug therapy but then I have to add in the increased risks associated with Tamoxifen. How would I make an equation out of that? Something with fractions and

variables? Would it involve probability theory? I feel
my math ineptitude coming back to haunt me. "I can't
wait to see what the nutritionist says," I say. "I'm going
to show her what I'm doing and she'll tell me what else
I can do."

The nutritionist is also an M.D. and an acupunctur-
ist, a lovely Indian woman with creamy almond-colored
skin and shiny black hair and a name that lilts as it rolls
off her tongue. I imagine she's descended from very
wise people, yogis and sages and I am ready to absorb
her wisdom, follow her orders whatever they may be.

I pull out my four-page list. "So this is what I have
been eating and these are the things I've been avoiding
and up until a couple of days ago, I thought I had it all
figured out. But then I read about plant estrogens and
borons and it turns out a lot of the *good* foods may actually be *bad* foods? And now I'm so confused I don't
know what to eat."

She glances at my list. "You actually follow these
rules and eat like this?"

I nod vigorously.

"Good for you. That's very impressive. There are
some 'bad' estrogens and you want to avoid them. Eating organic is one way. But plant estrogens? Let's type it
into the computer and see what we find." She Googles
Plant Estrogens. Up pop the sites I have read and practically memorized. She clicks on the first few and I watch
her read what I just told her and she turns to me and says,

"I say eat a variety of healthful foods and exercise and take the Tamoxifen and don't miss your mammograms."

"But what about the borons?" I ask.

She types *Borons.* . . . "From what I can see, there aren't any definitive studies on borons and breast cancer. So again, rotate your diet, eat as healthfully as you are and. . . . "

"What about parabens?"

"Parabens?"

"The stuff they put in shampoos and conditioners and lotions to emulsify them?"

"I don't know about parabens." Her lovely, strong fingers type *Parabens.* The Canadian study appears on the screen. "It looks like there was one study but it was pretty small. . . . "

"I've been avoiding them because that study showed traces of parabens in the breast tumors," I say. "Oh, and wine. I do have an occasional glass of wine even though I know that increases my risk slightly." I shuffle through my notes, but can't find the data. "But I figure it decreases my risk of stroke, which is increased from the Tamoxifen, so it probably evens out my overall health risk and I'm thinking it relaxes me which probably lowers my stress level . . . "

Her dark, penetrating eyes stare at me very intently as she nods her head.

". . . which could affect both my heart and my cancer risk. I read stress can cause cellular degradation and I *do* feel stressed. Marriage, kids, my career hasn't exactly taken off the way I'd hoped and then there's . . . the electromagnetic field. What do you think about the electromagnetic field? I work on a computer and last year we switched to wireless and in fact the whole world is practically wireless so now I've been thinking the field must be everywhere. Oh, and I almost forgot. I read a study that correlated lack of melatonin with an increased risk and I worry that I don't always sleep that soundly and now with the Tamoxifen which is known to cause insomnia I'm worried that could get worse and then there's a whole slew of data out there claiming Tamoxifen is *more* harmful than. . . . "

She clears her throat to interrupt me, turns the computer screen away from us and leans toward me and faces me squarely, rests her sturdy hands so close to mine I'm certain she's going to hold them and tell me exactly how to make sense of all this conflicting information.

"You've done an incredible job of researching all this," she says. "But, you can't live in a bubble. None of us can. You have a life and you should live it as fully as possible. Embrace every little bit of it. The stressors and the joy. Ride it like a roller coaster. We aren't sages— and even sages get cancer. But you are a smart and very determined woman and if you have to deal with recurrence or another surgery or whatever, you need to trust that you will do whatever it is you need to do to get through it."

I'm tearing up but sucking it in because although I know what she's saying is true and wise even, I'm waiting for . . . a Buddhist blessing, magical elixirs, dictums. Yes, a list of dictums that I would follow no matter how complicated or restrictive because I am willing to go to whatever lengths it takes . . . but that's it. She stops talking and I look down at the crumpled unanswered questions on the desk and feel like I did when I was twelve and realized my mother was not as powerful as I thought. No matter how hard I tried to go back to the illusion that she would always guide and safeguard me, I couldn't help but see that she was just a woman doing the best she could. I was on my own.

I stand and shake the nutritionist's hand and mumble thank you as I stuff my list back in my bag, shuffle out to the waiting room, and find Mike half dozing in a chair.

"So?" he says. "What did she say?"

I shrug and say real fast, "She said I'm doing everything I can."

"See?" he says and holds my hand. "You're going to be fine."

"One more biopsy and the tits are history." I make a chop-chop gesture and start marching toward the exit.

"She said that?"

"No. I didn't talk to her about that. She's a nutritionist."

"So what *did* she say?"

"I told you. She said I'm doing everything I can," I snap. "Take the Tamoxifen. Get my mammograms blah blah blah."

"What did you want?" he says, catching up beside me.

I say nothing as we walk down the wide venerable halls, past the Andy Warhols and the doctors huddling, past the plaque, and I wonder, What *did* I want?

We stop for the elevator and I turn to Mike and say, "I guess . . . I wanted . . . someone to tell me what to eat, to drink, how to breathe, where to put my foot. I wanted a . . . guarantee." As soon as the words cross my lips, I feel embarrassed for saying them. I know the truth: I have a bum breast with unpredictable cells and nobody knows what cancer has in store for me, and doctors (even the ones at Mayo) don't proffer guarantees.

[*sixteen*]

The Mother Who
Runs Up the Hill

I'M IN THE kitchen making another batch of organic face lotion. I've been thinking I'll start an organic facial products company, ever since the day my marital therapist said my skin was glowing and asked me what I was using on it. I gave him my whole parabens-are-toxic schpiel, explained that I was using only homemade products now, and he asked me if I would bring him some to try.

Mike thinks this is a phase. He reminds me of other phases I've gone through: the advertising executive phase; the stand-up comic and acting phase; the I'm going to save the poor Russian children at the Yeshiva phase, which morphed into the teaching in Hell's Kitchen phase; the going back to graduate school and wanting to be a professor phase; the Hemingway-inspired journalist phase; the why not be a local TV anchor phase; the law school phase that has been coming and going for more than twenty years; the Bikram Yoga teacher training phase I didn't pursue because it required too many months in L.A.

He thinks soon I'll be writing another novel. But he's wrong. First of all, I haven't been hearing much at all from my agent and I know our split is just a matter of one of us formally calling it quits. Secondly, the *only* thing I can write about is my diagnosis and its aftermath and all my crazy, obsessive thoughts, which I scribble in my journal furtively and plan *never* to show anyone.

And when I'm not writing in my journal, I'm studying *Natural Beauty at Home: More Than 250 Easy-to-Use Recipes for Body, Bath and Hair.* I plan to make all 250 and bottle the best ones and call the company Fraiche (because you have to make fresh batches every few days and keep them refrigerated) and market it to other vain hypochondriacal maniacs like me.

I'm stirring shea butter, jojoba oil, and grated beeswax into a pot when my fourth-grade son bursts into the kitchen, flushed and trying so hard not to cry it makes me want to cry.

"Adam said you were like, like . . . Tyler's mom."

I drop the spoon into the pot of hot oil and am unable to speak. Tyler's mother died of breast cancer a few years ago, leaving three school-aged boys and a shell-shocked husband.

"You know that's not true," I say. Still, I can't help but wonder if this is how my son perceives me, like Tyler's mother, just a matter of time.

"I told him they got all the cancer out and then I told him, 'My Mom's an athlete. She can run up all the hills in the neighborhood.'"

I gulp. I've been running, but barely. Plodding and panting and avoiding the hills. Spending most of my energy making lists of what *not* to eat, how to dodge toxins, whipping up batches and batches of all-natural beauty products and perhaps, most significantly, not truly believing I am or ever will be healthy enough to run like I used to.

Alex can't hold off the tears any longer. He's crying now and I'm hugging him and crying now, too, because I realize I was wrong about the slow fade. The slow fade is worse. He needs and wants me to be here and strong, and I want and need that too, more than anything, and I've been wasting precious time worrying, paralyzed by the thought of what might happen next.

I cup his warm, wet face in my hands and think, This is the worst part of this whole ordeal: to see me diminished in my son's eyes, to know that the loss of a mother (of me) would rock his foundation. Damn it. I hate myself, my cells, the weakness in me, the stress and strain I've dumped in our lives.

"Adam is wrong," I say. "I'm going to be fine."

He looks doubtful. And who can blame him? How can I win back his trust? How can I prove to him that I'm okay?

"You wanna arm wrestle?" I say and slap my elbow on the table.

He shrugs and then he clasps my hand and pretends to struggle against mine and lets me win.

"Next time I'll beat you fair and square," I tell him and ruffle his hair with my fingers and fake slug him.

He sniffles and wipes his tears with the back of his forearm and nods as I pick up the phone and with him still standing there, I call my best friend Martha and tell her I *will* run the Half-Marathon in NYC with her in August.

"I want to do speed work and cross-training and core strengthening and lots and lots of hills," I say, thinking, If nothing else, I will be the mother who can run up all the hills in the neighborhood.

When I hang up the phone, he finally cracks a little smile and says, "Game of hoops?"

seventeen

Cancer Snakes
Its Way Through
the Neighborhood

THE DAYS LENGTHEN and brighten and daffodils poke through the warming earth and cancer snakes its way through the neighborhood: a brain tumor on the corner of Oakwood; kidney next to the country club; early-stage prostate on the top of Chestnut Hill; inoperable lung behind the elementary school. The threat of death is everywhere and I wonder, Was it always there and I just didn't notice it? Like when I was pregnant and suddenly it seemed everyone was pregnant?

Only I don't want to notice death. I want to notice life and living. But I know, even if I'm lucky and this cancer thing leaves me alone, it's relentless, devastating other people's lives, people I don't even know well but I can't help but feel for. I'm part of a club I didn't mean to join.

Although honestly, most days I can't take the responsibility of being "The Woman Who Had Breast Cancer." It's hard work. Explaining the story, assuring people I'm okay and they're okay, then dealing with my very presence tweaking their fears about their own mortality, which in turn re-tweaks my own, an utterly exhausting cycle that often ends in my not wanting to go anywhere, and yet forcing myself to go everywhere people might expect me to be because I don't want them to think I'm not somewhere because I'm sick.

"You're the most health-conscious person I know," a neighbor says. "If it could happen to you, people think it could happen to them." I feel her studying me, wondering what I did wrong that she shouldn't do.

"Random bad luck," I tell her. "And since it hit me, I think your odds are better." I'm still not totally clear on how this odds thing works, but she walks away looking a little relieved.

Another friend tells me that every time she gets upset about anything now her husband says, "'What are you complaining about—it's not like you've had cancer or anything.' Oh God, I shouldn't be telling you this, should I?" she says.

"Are you kidding?" I say. "Life can suck even if you aren't worried about your health."

"Well," she says. "At least you don't have to worry about Anya [a mutual friend of ours] not liking you."

"Anya didn't like me?"

"Um . . . not really, but now she *does* because she doesn't want to be you anymore."

Maybe I can try denial. Denial sounds good to me. When I was growing up we lived in a very Christian and Catholic neighborhood. I could "pass" for Italian or Irish and even though I felt guilty about it, I often didn't tell people I was Jewish. It was easier. I can walk into the Silent Auction and Ice Cream Social with my son and pretend "it" never happened. I'm walking. I'm smiling. I'm Greek. I'm Spanish. I'm Yoda. I'm a Space Cowboy. I'm placing bids. Watching Alex eat a great big Blue Moon ice cream cone and as I'm leaving, a woman I barely know, who I heard is convinced she has ovarian cancer because of the neighborhood scares, pulls me over and says, "Did you know they can suck your uterus right out of your vagina?"

In mid-April, Anna is accepted at Bard College and we're all thrilled and relieved and wonder why we ever cared about Dartmouth. I throw myself into planning Anna's graduation party, which we decide will be in the backyard filled with flowers and all her favorite finger foods and music piping out of the living room, French doors flung open wide, a party so fabulous that it would make Mrs. Hart proud. I'd always pictured us having more of those spontaneous-looking parties you see in glossy magazines, where everything looks simple but elegant, including the hostess. But now I wonder, Have I thrown enough parties?

When the kids were little I loved planning birthday parties for them; making homemade cakes that always tasted better than they looked and homemade invitations covered in too much glitter, tossing peanuts in the lawn for a peanut hunt, hanging piñatas to be smashed and donkeys to be tailed. The year Mike started earning a salary that finally covered our living expenses was the year Anna turned five and we celebrated by going to Target and buying all the birthday party crap we couldn't afford before, including so many party treats for the guests that I had to make special goodie bags out of taped-together tissue paper to hold the loot.

But the day was too hot and Anna so overwhelmed by her own party that by the time we walked outside with the already sagging triple-layered chocolate chocolate cake singing "Happy Birthday," she was dripping in sweat and burst into tears. When I did start throwing "grown-up" parties, they didn't feel the way I expected them to. There were the Dinner Party Years for Mike's colleagues and Mike always saying, "Just tell me what to do," and then disappearing and I'd find him changing all the storm windows, when I'd asked him to go buy a bag of ice. By the time the guests arrived we'd be fighting. So the whole party-throwing thing hasn't exactly been our strength.

But. This party for Anna is going to be different from all those parties. This party will celebrate all that Anna is and will be and the pure wondrousness of life and living. How could it not be, with the hardy roses and miniature hydrangea trees in bloom? It's spring! A time of renewal! The life-force exerting itself! Everything healthy and new!

Every night, after I go over the list of things I still need to do for the party, I pray for my newly diagnosed neighbors and their families and then I pray that the results of my six-month checkup in July don't require more surgery and distract me from getting Anna settled in college in the fall. The fall needs to be about her. Just give us that, God. Just that.

I call my mother to invite her to the party and she says, "I'd love to come but I'm speaking at a conference in Boca Raton that weekend."

My mother, who became an occupational therapist later in life, after many degrees (including philosophy and literature and theater), has recently become a leading authority on Parkinson's disease, having developed a ground-breaking therapy. I'm delighted that she's finally found her calling and is being recognized. I think a large part of her frustration as a wife and mother was that my dad's ambition left no room for her own. She was too brainy and unconventional to play devoted and adoring lawyer's wife and suburban mother of four, especially in the '60s and '70s. I often think she shouldn't have had children at all and I imagine meeting her as my bright, funny, eccentric neighbor and really liking her.

"That's okay," I say, thinking her *and* my dad and my stepmother visiting all at once would probably be too much.

"Did I tell you my favorite nun is praying for you?" she asks.

"I think you wrote that in your last card," I say. "The one with all the angels."

"Did I tell you I wish I could be a nun?"

See, this is what I'm talking about. As her neighbor/friend, this is funny stuff. As her daughter, slightly more disturbing than funny.

"No, you didn't," I say.

"Well, I do," she says. "That or a saint."

"You're doing good work, Mom," I say. She is and I know she hasn't been told that enough.

"Oh honey, you're so darling. I love talking to you. I'm so glad we're getting close again."

We're all in the backyard, under a red and white striped tent that doesn't exactly go with the party color scheme but we had to rent it at the last minute because we woke to an early June drizzle, when my dad and stepmother, who had her own breast cancer scare a decade ago, arrive two hours into Anna's graduation party. I haven't seen them in a couple of years, and I always turn thirteen and a little chubby and a lot awkward and unsure of who I am, *if* I am.

My stepmother came into my life when I was twelve and hurt and angry and confused by my parents' divorce. She was young and glamorous with big blond hair and those big boobs and a stomach that was flatter than mine and unusually pretty hands that she adorned with funky rings and bracelets, and she and my dad were determined to have fun while my mother was unraveling. The thing is, she was twenty-eight and really did adore my dad, but I don't think she was mature enough to handle the whole package, the four kids, the messy complications.

She didn't understand the power of her impact on us. And I was the most outspoken, the one always in their faces. When she told my little sister (who was six at the time) that it was weird that she wanted to sit next to my dad on the hump in the car at her age, I told my stepmother she was cruel and crazy. And I told my dad that he was a coward not to stand up to her. Which didn't go over so well.

I was an easy target. Not a standout in any way (other than my blunt candor): not athletic; not a great student (before the divorce I had been, but after, I didn't care); not a great beauty (people said I had a pretty face but I was chubby so you had to look for it). Most of my friends in high school were the kids from the other side of the railroad tracks who liked to smoke in the parking lot and skip school.

Of course, deep down I wanted my dad and step-mother to adore me anyway. Like my friend Susie Day, who was tall and gawky and certainly not a brain, but every time her parents saw her, they lit up as if she were a movie star. When I walked into a room, my dad and stepmom could barely hide their discomfort and disappointment, their desire for me to disappear.

The year they had a son (my half-brother, Sam) was the year I went away to college (at sixteen). I started slimming down and regaining confidence. I wrote poetry and was published; I created a women's literary magazine, wrote a thesis, racked up a few more publications, and spoke on a writers' panel, while graduating with honors.

I remember the day I excitedly brought my thesis over to show them: I handed it to my stepmother and dad, thinking now they would see that I was someone, but they distractedly flipped through it, then tossed it on the coffee table just in time for my half-brother, who was five then, to slap a sticky hand on the cover page and rip it.

After graduation, my aimless years in New York City, I flitted from advertising to acting to waitressing to teaching, from one dark, brooding indecisive boyfriend to the next, showing no real promise professionally or personally. It wasn't until the day I introduced them to Mike that they took notice of me. They were visiting NYC from Ohio and I'd told them I wanted to introduce them to my new boyfriend. I felt their admiration of him as soon as we walked into the restaurant.

Mike's clean-cut, Aryan looks mesmerized and intimidated and maybe even slightly alarmed them. He shook their hands and politely asked them about their flight and then the conversation turned to Dartmouth and his junior year abroad and Rugby and skiing and tennis and his plans for medical school. I knew they couldn't figure out what he was doing with me, but it made them look at me, really look at me for the first time. And although this is very embarrassing to admit, not very modern womanish, I thought, If he claims me, maybe they'll finally want to claim me, too.

We'd expected them to arrive at Anna's party much earlier but they like to be late. Who can blame them? The last time my dad visited a couple of years before was a bit of a disaster. After too much small talk, including a lengthy and detailed analysis by my stepmother about the inadequacies of the restaurant we had taken them to the night before, I asked my dad to go for a walk with me, surprising myself with the request.

Outside I said, "You leaving us . . ." I choked. ". . . destroyed my childhood and my self-esteem and I think the reason Daniel. . . ." Then I burst into tears.

And he said, "Your mother was crazy. I couldn't live with her."

"Then why did you leave us with her? How could you?"

He shrugged and I shuddered as tears streamed down my face. He put his arm around me and hugged me and I felt like he finally understood. I thought, Now I can ask him all the questions I'd been wanting to ask about Daniel. Like did he really believe he was schizophrenic or did he think it was just a bad psychotic episode caused by depression perhaps brought on by all the family dysfunction. I could tell him about a book I'd read called *How to Become a Schizophrenic* that explained so much to me and how while I understood it made him feel better as a parent to think Daniel's problem was organically based, it made me as a parent feel *more* frightened and could we just agree that it might *not* have been schizophrenia?

But before I could articulate any of that, he said, "I gave you something. Now you have to give me something."

"What?"

"Tell me you understand I did what I had to do."

We were standing in the middle of my street and I was shaking and weeping for all my neighbors to see and even though I didn't mean it, I mumbled, "I understand." Just to end it. We headed back inside and I felt like an idiot.

Now, I spot his bald head and crinkly forehead and his thick gray beard. Was it *that* gray last time? And my stepmother in her dyed-blond halo and flowy dress. When did she get so old and shapeless? They're chatting with my yoga teacher, Rita, who I still think could be really good for Mike, and my best friend Martha, who is wearing a sleeveless dress with a black and white skull motif, and my hairdresser, Jay, who also is an elevator repairman, an electrician, a landscaper, musician, and friend. He built his own sound studio in his basement, next to the hairdressing room, and he and Anna arranged and cut a CD last year that she included in her college application package, her voice so tender and poignant it gave me shivers. I see Mike seeing me see my dad and he walks over and places his hand on the small of my back.

"Wow," my Dad says after making his way through the crowd, surveying the party. "You have a lot of . . . interesting friends."

I'm not sure how to take that and while my instinct would be to explain who everybody was and try to impress them with further explanations, make excuses for any flaws like the mismatched circus tent, I take another look around at the little pots of violets and the trays of bruchettas and finger sandwiches and Anna's favorite chocolate-dipped macaroons. I hear "Crimson and Clover," which Anna and I recently discovered both of us love, our youths dovetailing for a song, and I find Anna smiling and sure as she mingles between her friends and mine. And I'm completely bowled over by her beauty and strength, by the woman she has managed to blossom into, in spite of me and my shortcomings.

I find Alex laughing in the tree fort with the other boys and Maddy chatting giddily with her circle in the driveway and I take note of all our wonderful, quirky and not-so-quirky friends. I'm struck by how many people we have in our lives who we really know and care about, and it occurs to me I don't give a shit what my dad or my stepmother thinks.

I know what I think. I am here, thank God. And this is my house, my family, my garden, my life and what I have and don't have is all of my own accord and I don't need them or Mike or anyone to claim me. I need to claim myself.

"And they say such great things about you. . . . " My dad's still talking, I realize.

"How much did you pay them?" my stepmother jokes.

"And Mike and the kids," my dad says, barely missing a beat. "Everyone looks great."

"Anna is stunning," my stepmother says. "And you're . . . all grown up," she says.

"I'm forty-five," I say.

She laughs. "That's right. I always think you're sixteen. But you're so thin," she says, words I longed to hear at sixteen but now sound more critical than complimentary.

"I lost a little weight because I've been . . . "—I think about but don't mention my *Keys To NOT Being That*

12% (which I crossed out and switched to *14%*) list—
". . . training for a half-marathon," I say.

"Really, huh? I gained weight on Tamoxifen. You sure you're okay?"

Here it is, our bond, the thought of our mutated cells intertwined like twisted soul sisters maddening me. In a flood I see every rolled eye, every curled lip, hear every snide remark she made about my body, my hair, my thoughts, my taste in books and movies and men, my inadequacies in every department that mattered to her, the hours I listened to them wax poetic about all the "other people" who were more accomplished, more worthy than me and while I wanted them to "see" me, to "get" me, to love me, I never wanted to be the person their judgment would have created.

The truth is, they don't even know me. To them I'm Mike's wife. Anna, Maddy, and Alex's mother. Nothing more. This is my sole accomplishment in the world and more than they ever expected from me.

But I put all that aside and answer the question. "I'm okay. They're keeping a very close eye on me. Thanks for asking," I say.

"Well, that's good to know," she says and tilts her head and smiles.

And even though I'm . . . let's say shocked, I think I detect more concern than criticism and I take that in and smile back at her.

After most of the guests leave, Rita, my yoga teacher, leads Mike and Alex and his friends in yoga stretches and omming in the family room while my hairdresser, Jay, and his wife talk politics with my dad and stepmother in the dining room.

"I want the same exact party for my graduation in two years," Maddy says to me at the sink in the kitchen.

"That good, huh?" I say and hand her another glass to dry.

"Yeah, that good," Anna pipes in and squeezes in on the other side of me.

I'm so happy, my body wedged between my girls at the sink, my house buzzing with lively chatter—our tribute to Anna with a nod to Mrs. Hart—that I'm nearly choking on the absolute fullness of this moment when I say, "Okay, same party year after next."

Then I realize I need an extension on the *just getting through the fall* for Anna. I want to get through Maddy's graduation and Anna's college graduation and then Alex's graduation and then Anna's first job and Maddy's first job and Alex's college graduation and all their first jobs and marriages and grandchildren and. . . .

A few weeks later, we're packing the car with Maddy's kayaking and camping equipment—sleeping bag, sleep pad, wetsuit, thermal wear, paddling gloves, sunblock, waterproof camera, first-aid kit—and are just about to leave the house to drive Maddy to camp, when the phone rings and I hear that Dawn Myers, the woman I ran into at the airport, has been diagnosed with colon cancer, already metastasized, and she is picking up her distraught daughter from camp early.

I can't believe it. It isn't possible. I just saw her. At the airport. She was fine. She's a runner. She's healthy. She's smart. She's funny. She giggles . . . and, and it's summer and everything is in bloom. This must be wrong wrong wrong.

"What's the matter?" Mike asks me as I crouch in the bathroom, the dial tone from the dropped phone echoing between my knees.

I mumble something but my thoughts are so disjointed, I'm not sure what I've said.

"I'm sorry," he says, kneeling down beside me. "That sounds serious. That's sad."

I nod and bury my head in my hands and say, "But she could still be okay. Right?" I nod. "She could survive this. Right?" I nod. "People survive. Right?" I nod. "She's a fighter."

He nods a tiny bit, pats my hand and stands and tries to pull me up by my arm. "We have to take Maddy to camp now."

"What about the life preserver?" I say.

"What?" he says.

"She needs a life jacket," I say.

"The camp provides them. Remember?"

He kneels down again and gently helps me up and this time I rise up and into his arms and he hugs me and says, "You're going to be okay."

"I'm not talking about me," I say, leaning into his chest.

"I know," he says, petting my head. "Let's go."

The whole trip, a trip we've taken many times, with Anna all the years she went to camp, that traditionally involves the girls introducing me to their music and lots of loud chatting about friend and teacher troubles and the roadkill game to amuse Alex and a stop at our favorite coffee and ice cream shop halfway (but this time it's just Maddy and Mike in the car, the other children with friends for the day) and I weep silently as I slither inside Dawn and her daughter's skin, writhing back and forth between imagining how it must feel to be the mother picking up her daughter, to be the daughter of the sick mother.

eighteen

My Oncologist
Isn't Happy

LAKEVIEW HAS MOVED oncology to a building separate from the rest of the clinic. At my last appointment, I passed pediatrics and obstetrics and dermatology, waiting rooms filled with younger patients. Now, I enter the lobby with the old, the bald, the sallow skinned, the decrepit, jogging past them in my yoga pants, taking the stairs two by two.

The receptionist asks me if I'm here to pick up my mother.

I shake my head. "No. I have a 2:00 with Dr. Bromowitz."

"You look just like Mrs. Arnold's daughter."

"People always say I look like someone," I say, thinking I wish I *were* Mrs. Arnold's daughter, and take a seat and wait my turn.

In the examining room, my oncologist walks in with my chart and drops it on the desk with a flourish. He's pissed. He shakes his head as he ruffles through the pages. "I've gone over the slides, talked to the pathologist [George] and I stand by the original diagnosis—DCIS, intermediate grade." He starts drawing some squiggly lined pictures, using the words "spectrum" and "mutation" and "cellular integrity." "How's the Tamoxifen going? Hot flashes? Weight gain? Bloating? Insomnia?" he says.

I shake my head. "I feel great!" I say, hoping that will make him happier.

"Just wait," he says and shrugs. "Sit over there." He points to the examination table. "Take your shirt off."

I get up and walk over to the table and hop on and kind of shake my head and say, "They did a *very* thorough breast exam at Mayo—the doctor, her assistant, *and* a med student. And Nancy [my breast surgeon] also examined them a few weeks ago. Maybe you don't need to?"

"Take your shirt off," he says again, standing right up next to me.

I feel strange about taking my shirt off without a gown but he's standing so close and I feel intimidated by his hulking presence, so I pull my shirt over my head and unsnap and remove my bra.

I take a deep breath as he presses his fingers on my breasts in the most cursory way and then examines them with his eyes and I see them as he must: asymmetrical, slashed with scars that haven't faded. "Still dense," he says. "I'll see you in a month." And he storms out of the examining room, the air from the opened door chilling my bare flesh.

As soon as I find my car and unlock the door and buckle myself in, the strap pulling taut against my chest, I picture the oncologist, his angry face, his hand on my breasts, think about a worm I accidentally squished in the parking lot on the way to my car, and my shoulders collapse into the steering wheel.

At the grocery store, a few weeks later, I fill my cart with organic grapes and berries, peaches and plums, raw walnuts, almonds, dark chocolate, green tea, and fresh whole-grain seduction bread along with a meditation-for-healing DVD and *Body and Soul* magazine. I also toss in tissue paper, a card, and a wicker basket, and back in my car I wrap and arrange everything, then drive it over to Dawn's house and leave it just inside the vestibule.

She calls me a day later and thanks me for the basket and I ask her if she'd like to go for a walk.

That afternoon, I meet her in front of her house, a little afraid. I know she started chemo and I'm not sure what to expect. I'm staring down at my sneakers, bracing myself, when she comes bouncing out the front door dressed adorably in shorts and a little t-shirt, her fit little teenager body, her lovely reddish hair still lovely, her eyes sparkling, her smile as wide as ever. She doesn't look any different than last time I saw her, in fact she might even look better. More alive.

I remember the first time I met her a few years back on the running trail, she was training for a triathlon and had just completed a half-mile swim in the lake and she joined Martha and me for a run. She was having a hard time keeping up that day and it surprised me since we weren't going all that fast and I'd always thought of her as much more of an athlete than me. That day I thought it was probably because she swam too hard before the run, but now I wonder if the cancer had already started gnawing away at her.

"Ready?" she says, all peppy as if we're starting a race.

I nod and we walk down the curvy hill toward the lake, past perfectly groomed boxwood hedges and showy perennial beds and empty recycling bins, and she asks me to tell her exactly what happened with my breast scare. So I go back to my first scare five years ago and give her my whole history, including the recent Mayo visit, my newly increased risk factor, my last oncology visit, the hormone therapy, and tell her I have my six-month checkup at the end of the month.

"It's nothing compared to what you're going through," I say, as we round the bottom of the country club, the bright-green grass blanket nearly blinding me in the afternoon sun. "I don't want to pry but do you want to talk about it?"

Then she tells me her story, the diagnosis, the shock, how she's started chemo and how it hasn't really affected her physically yet. "In fact, I feel fine!" she says.

"You look terrific," I say.

"I feel good," she says, her voice rising up.

We reach Lake Mendota Drive and the breeze from the lake is blowing our hair, obscuring our faces as we turn toward one another and I say, "You don't deserve this. It isn't fair."

She nods and then she says, "I'm actually happier than I've ever been." She tucks her hair behind her ears. "Everything is. . . . " She looks at me. Pauses.

"A little clearer and sharper, more intense?"

She nods.

"With unexpected moments of pure exhilaration thrown in?"

Keeps nodding.

"Like every day you wake up and think, This is it. This is my life. Everything matters."

"Yes, yes, that's it," she says. "Exactly." She smiles at me. "It's so great to talk to you about this."

We both glance across the lake.

"It's a gorgeous day. Isn't it?" she says.

"Glorious," I say and nod.

She stops then completely. We've been walking up a slight incline and I see she is a little winded and parched. "Did you bring water?" I ask her.

She shakes her head.

"Here." I hand her my water bottle and she takes a good, long swig and says, "Wow, that's good. Thank you!"

"Even water is better, huh?"

"Water is great," she says and then she giggles, just like a little girl and I love that about her—the little girl still in there—and then, I feel a flash of terror pass between us.

I'm tempted to clasp her hands in mine, but I don't know her that well and she doesn't seem like the hand-clasping type, but I look deep into her wide eyes and say, "You are one of the strongest, most vital women I know. You are going to beat this."

She nods, takes another swig of water and then we turn back around and as I walk her home, she's slowing, the outing has tired her much more than she's letting on and the whole way back I silently pray: She will survive, she will survive, she will survive.

It's the night of the annual Third of July Firemen's Dance and my t-shirt dress is sticking to my sweaty back as I stand outside the firehouse with my friend Polly, who is a pothead, but also (perhaps surprisingly to some) ambitious and responsible and fit, an all-around wonderful person who happens to like to get high. She's tried to get me to smoke with her, and I haven't, not because I think it's so bad but because I hate smoke and I'm afraid I'll get caught.

We're sharing wine out of her flask (from the pre-dance cocktail party at our friends' house nearby) and listening to the D.J. lead the dancers in the Macarena inside and the cicadas serenade the children in the field across the street playing flashlight tag without flashlights, squealing in near hysteria, as we discuss Dawn and the neighborhood cancer scares and the whole cosmic weirdness of the first half of this year. Polly's great to talk to when she's stoned, reminds me of being in college and staying up all night and pondering the essence of dust.

Last year I remember standing here with Dawn and explaining to her the reason I didn't like this dance was because it was a microcosm of the neighborhood social hierarchy. I pointed out the pecking order and the scheming I had already witnessed, and Dawn laughed at my interpretation of the dance and said she'd never noticed any of that; and I thought, That's because she's a brilliant scientist with much more important things on her mind.

"We should get Dawn stoned," I whisper in Polly's ear now.

She laughs. "I can't believe you're saying that."

"In California it's medically sanctioned. You watch *Weeds*, right?"

She shakes her head. "No. I've never seen that show but if you think it would make her feel better, sure. I'm all for it. So you wanna just pop over there now?"

I kind of do, but then I see it: us at Dawn's house sitting cross-legged in her living room, smoking a joint and the police bust in and we're handcuffed and thrown in jail. The headline: MAPLEWOOD MOTHERS CAUGHT TOKING splashed across the front page of the local paper.

"I don't know her well enough to just pop over," I say. "And maybe not tonight. But soon. . . . "

"Sure," Polly says and rolls her eyes and we both turn toward a clutch of the tall, good-looking men pounding beer and discussing strategies for the next day's water fight against the firemen. I think about the cute blond mom who got drunk and jumped a fireman at the end of the night a couple of years back. I wasn't there and I don't think anything happened beyond that, but I loved that Cute Blond Mom was still so in touch with her wild side and found new respect for her.

Polly offers me more wine from her flask as a brainy researcher neighbor guy approaches the aggressively vivacious ex-president of the Village League behind us and says, "Did you know that scientists recently discovered the earth has rotated a fraction of an inch?"

Village League ignores Researcher Guy and flexes her taut tennis arms and bats her eyes at the best looking of the Good-Looking Men who is entranced by his re-filled beer.

"Did you hear that?" Polly says to me. "Cosmic forces altering the cosmos." She offers me more wine as my son and his friends come roaring and bombing across the street and he smashes into my legs. He tells me he's heading inside to get a good spot for "Bye-Bye, Miss American Pie," and I glance back at the field emptying, the fireflies blinking against the dark canvas sky, faintly illuminating everything in general but nothing in particular.

"But if you think about it, in the scope of the earth's diameter it really isn't *that* big," Researcher Guy is saying to Village League who is still pining for Best-Looking Guy who is lovingly licking the foamy edges of his beer cup, everyone flirting and flexing with unrequited zeal. I imagine Dawn here, laughing and shaking her head at my interpretation and all at once it feels as if my nerve endings are so ignited they might burst out of my skin and set the whole world in flames. And I wonder, Is this how it feels to be fully alive or is this the specter of death coursing through my veins?

"Is he kidding?" I say more to myself than to Polly as she pulls me into the firehouse. "A fraction of an inch means that the space that separates humans, the sky from the earth, light from dark has shifted and that,

that would explain . . . everything." I wave my hands
overhead.

"You would be so fun stoned," Polly whispers in my
ear as we approach the edge of the dance floor and find
Alex and Mike and join them in the final song of the
night, as we all sing Bye-Bye to Miss American Pie.

nineteen

My Health
Is the
Dining Room Table

IWANT TO go back to Anna's graduation party and stand at the kitchen sink, securely wedged between my girls, Alex and Mike's laughter glazing the air, and wade in our quintessence forever. I want more *now* but life keeps hurtling forward in spite of what I want. My six-month checkup is next week and even though I haven't been obsessing as much about my health, now every night I lie in bed flipping back and forth between hoping everything will be okay and fearing it won't.

Mike wraps his thigh over my thigh but I feel too hot and sticky and try to wiggle free as I say, "I'm thinking if I can just get the right handle on how to think about my fears then I can ward them off."

He repositions his leg and stares at the ceiling.

"I'm aware this is magical thinking," I say. "It's not like I'm completely out of my mind but if you think about it, isn't life full of magical thinking? I mean the fact that we get up every day and get dressed and step out the door as if loss isn't lurking right around the corner just waiting to flatten us?"

He swats a nonexistent gnat and props himself up on his elbows and clears his throat and I think he's going to say something. But he doesn't. His silence reminds me of my dad and stepmother's silence as if anything I had to say was so insignificant that it didn't warrant a response.

I want more from Mike. More from life. But is more too much? Am I too much? Too intense? Too sensitive? Too temperamental? Too too too?

Would he be happier with one of those cooler, more restrained wives? Sometimes I think he would, when I'm not thinking he'd be happier with Rita, my yoga teacher, who could relax him, or Laura New Hampshire, who could organize him. Maybe one of each depending on his mood, but in this moment I think restrained is what he'd like. . . .

I try to restrain myself. But I don't.

"Do you think I should have an elective mastectomy even if the mammogram is fine?" I say, instead.

I've been thinking about this more and more. Wondering why I don't have the elective surgery, and asking all my friends for their advice. Most said they'd get rid of the boobs. And I would too, if it didn't involve surgery. One of my friends put me in touch with her sister who'd just had a double mastectomy and reconstruction and I called her and she was so upbeat and cheery and said the surgery wasn't too bad and that she was up and running (literally, she's a runner, too) in a couple of weeks and that week she was scheduled for tattoos. And I thought, Wow, she really *is* handling this well. Breast surgery and tattoos in such a short period of time. She's *much* cooler and hipper than I am. I was about to ask her what she was planning to have tattooed and where, when she said, "They won't look exactly like my nipples but the color of the tattoo is pretty close." And then I was grabbing and clutching my breasts. I hadn't thought the surgical implications through that far and the reality of losing and replacing that part of my body seemed much more drastic than I'd imagined. I shared a little of this with Mike but I stopped when I saw that it was even harder for him to hear.

"I'm not sure," Mike finally says now.

"Do you think it will come back more aggressively?"

"I'm not sure but I think we should buy a new couch for the family room. The one we have has been through too many surgeries."

"So you're saying you think I'm going to be okay?"

"I don't know but I saw this great down couch at Vintage Door. If we order it now, we can have it in two months."

I'm annoyed by this couch talk. Annoyed because I know this is his way of thinking he can buy us out of uncertainty. In marital therapy, Mike and I learned that his father's refusal to buy his mother the dining room table she wanted was a major symbol of the dysfunction in their marriage and the reason why Mike was absolutely determined to earn enough money so he would never have to deny his wife the thing she wanted most. The reason why earning money and having money took priority over almost every other aspect of our lives to the point where I have screamed on more than one occasion that I don't give a shit about the money.

One time we were driving to Florida when the girls were small and Mike was a resident and we hadn't been on vacation in three years and I rarely got out of the house and couldn't remember the last time we'd talked about anything other than practical matters. I told him how lonely I was for adult company. For marriage.

"Do you know how many women would love to switch places with you?" he said.

"Why, because you're a doctor?"

He nodded smugly. "And you're not getting any younger," he said.

I felt slapped. "I'd rather live with an auto mechanic who lived in a trailer . . . " I pointed to a trailer park just off the exit, "who talked to me and rubbed my feet at night than. . . . "

He swerved to the side of the road so abruptly our wheels skidded sideways on the gravel edge. "Get out!" he said. "Who do you think would want you with two small children anyway? Have you looked at yourself recently? Your looks aren't what they used to be."

It was true. I knew it was true. I was a mother and so devoted to that role that I'd lost the woman in me. My entire being a vessel for other people's needs. But I wanted to leave. I wanted to open the car door and step over the guardrail, across the scrubby, trash-strewn brush and into another life, the life I'd meant to be living. But it was the middle of nowhere and the girls were in the car. I had no money and I couldn't think where I would go or who I would call (my parents would think I was crazy to leave "the doctor," and the few friends I'd kept in touch with had their own problems).

I'm not proud to admit this, but I didn't open the door. Instead I leaned over and hissed (so the girls wouldn't hear), "Fuck you," and climbed over the seat, into the back, where I wedged myself between the girls' car seats, and we drove on—and I felt like a coward.

When we got back home from that trip, I couldn't figure out what to do. How to take control of my life without turning into my mother and causing irreparable damage to my children. I reasoned staying was a way to right the wrongs of my childhood. And people who say they don't stay for the children—they're lying. I'm not saying people only stay for the children but I know there were many lulls and nasty fights and if not for the look of despair I imagined on their faces, I would have walked. And never looked back.

But the money? I didn't stay for the money. The money has been much more of a problem than a pleasure for me. It has given Mike the upper hand. Made him think he could dictate how we lived, but I didn't protest enough. I wasn't brave or strong enough to figure out what I deserved and every time I mentioned marital therapy, he said he'd *never* share the details of our private life with a stranger. . . . It took ten more years and me yearning so desperately for the me I had buried that I found *myself* in such despair that I walked out the door and spent the whole night in the car listening and crying to Bonnie Raitt's "I Can't Make You Love Me," over and over and over again.

By dawn I figured I had nothing to lose. This wasn't love. This wasn't marriage. This was two people existing side by side, biding time until their lives really began. I walked back in that morning and said, "You either come to therapy with me or I'm leaving you."

And he did, although he said almost nothing for the first year and during that time, when I was alone with the therapist, I asked him how long this process would take, how long I should wait. "I'm not getting younger," I kept saying. "I want more." And the therapist said, "When Alex turns ten, if it isn't better, you can leave."

Alex turned ten this year. Two months after my breast surgery. And while I hadn't thought about what the therapist said in a couple of years and while our marriage *has* improved, still the timing strikes me now.

And the thing Mike still doesn't get is I *never* wanted a dining room table. Or a new couch. His mother wanted the damn table and he's spent most of his life trying to please his mother, thinking what she wanted is what all generic women want and utterly confused by the fact that my needs are not her needs. The things I want, I've told him, many times, in therapy and out, can't be bought.

I want a deep and abiding companionship and part-nership. I want each of us to be the soft spot for the other to land on, I want our home and our family to nurture and enrich all of us, I want our level of trust to be so solid that we can laugh and cry out loud, with our entire being. I want us to feel open and free to be our best selves and now I want my health. But he can't buy that either, can't give me what I want, and that makes him feel utterly powerless as a physician and a husband.

My health is the dining room table and we've suc-ceeded in reliving his parents' marriage in spite of six years of intensive therapy. And right now, right now I want his mother and her damn table and my dad and stepmother and their silences and my mother and her inability to be a woman and a mother simultaneously to leave our marriage and go home. It's way too crowded and confusing in here.

But I don't say any of that because the dining room table and the money and the power issues have been discussed and analyzed too many times to no avail and right now I don't have the energy for another fruitless battle. Instead, I want to use my energy to obsess about my upcoming appointment.

So I say, "Two months? I can't think about two months from now. It makes me feel superstitious and if you think about it, plans are kind of arrogant. Pre-sumptuous. I assume I can have coffee and chat with you in two weeks because NOTHING bad will happen to me to prevent it? Huh! Well, we both know *that* assumption isn't true."

Mike looks at me cockeyed and I wish I could stop myself from saying things that only add to his discomfort. I wish I could go back to a simpler time, when I tried to hide the inner me, the flaws, the ambiguity, the reckless desires, and be the wife who wanted to please him, who changed her hair and clothes and learned to ski (only after I told him I *could* ski and then we went skiing together and I freaked out at the top of the black diamond and fell and rolled most of the way down, losing the car keys) and cook and entertain and smile when I didn't want to and mother his children and move to the suburbs, even though I couldn't stand trying to fit into a life that wasn't me, that was *his* dream, *his* vision, *his* way. . . .

"All I want to know is if you think it's coming back," I say now. "I just feel like if I don't think this through and stay vigilant. . . . "

"You have to stop worrying so much," he says. "Most likely your checkup will be fine."

". . . although the damage was likely done years ago anyway," I say.

"What damage?" he asks a little defensively and I know he's thinking I'm talking about our marriage.

"The cellular damage?" I say. "Isn't that what one of those doctors told us? It doesn't happen overnight. So I've been thinking all my concern about my diet, well, I can see the irony of me, the health freak, getting struck again."

"Why do you say stuff like that?"

"Because it feels better to say what I fear than to think it and not say it. Isn't that what we learned in therapy?" I kick all the covers off and roll sideways, hoping this will relieve the heat rising in my body. "Do you feel like you're a moving target and no matter what you do it's likely you're gonna get hit anyway?"

He swats another gnat I can't see. "No, I don't," he says and sighs.

And I feel alone in my craziness. Or is it in my marriage? How can you ache for the person lying so close to you that you know and anticipate every sound, every move their body is capable of making, feel the pulse that permeates their skin permeate and alter your own as if their feelings are your feelings and it's hard to say where you begin and they end, where you end and they begin?

All the threads, the gaps and seams, interweaving webs that comfort on the verge of strangulation. The therapist told us we had boundary issues. But boundary schmoundary, how do you love without merging and mushing and blurring the edges? It isn't that my marriage is so bad now. In many ways I think we've survived the worst of it. We've been through so much together, birth and the threat of death, ecstasy and rage and everything in between.

I love him. I hate him. I want him. I don't. But why doesn't anyone tell you how risky it is to trust another person with the all of you, to imprint your life with their life? How frightening it is to love and let yourself be loved? That to stay with someone you have to get over and get on and be willing to redefine the marriage over and over again. And compromise. Always compromise.

It's like a peace treaty being negotiated over and over again. And how often marriage plays out like a Greek Tragedy, the timing just a bit off, each of your best intentions misfiring, your life stages out of sync? And why, after twenty years of marriage, does it feel as if in some ways we're strangers? How much do you really know about the person you share a life with?

I'm pretty sure we've both been faithful, but do I really know? When Mike was still an intern, and I was home with Anna and pregnant with Maddy, we had a party for the residents, and this resident doctor who was his supervisor showed up with a homemade strawberry rhubarb pie—his favorite—and they spent most of the night chuckling over beers in the corner.

I tried not to make a big deal out of it but I remembered that this was the woman who, he'd told me, had guided his hand while she performed surgery, letting him feel exactly what she knew. And I thought, They're closer than we are and possibly ever will be, and later that night and many times since I asked him if he slept with her. He always said no, he just really admired and respected her.

And that hurt me more than if he'd said they'd had a quick fuck because I wasn't sure he felt that way about me. Which is probably why I fell for a writer several years back whom I hired to help me edit my first novel. He said he loved my work and my voice, and I couldn't get enough of his praise and developed a crazy schoolgirl crush on him that reminded me of the first time I'd ever been kissed—that hot, sweet surprise—and everything was more vibrant and vivid and brimming with what could be.

We never met and after I realized how addicted I was to our interactions—and that I was essentially paying him to make me feel this way—I cut it off and told Mike. And he dismissed it, even though he'd always been jealous of old boyfriends I'd forgotten and men I hadn't noticed, but I'm sure it was because the guy was a poor, struggling artist and didn't seem like a threat. And I cried. Cried because I realized I'd conjured up feelings to fill an emptiness I hadn't realized the depth of until he filled it and cried because I'd been closed off and numb for so long when I longed to be open, to feel my feelings fully—but mostly I cried because I knew I would never leave my marriage and my life would likely never brim again.

"I know I sound crazy," I say now. "But you know I never used to worry about my health. I always thought I'd bounce back. From anything. Until this . . . I felt sturdy. Invincible. I did. But now I wonder if it was my cavalier attitude that got me in trouble with 'The Gods.'"

Mike rests his elbow on my hip and says, "Don't be silly. You know that's not true. You didn't do anything to make this happen and we're going to make sure you're going to be fine." His voice rising and cracking like a little boy's. Making me feel like a little girl and I wonder if either of us will grow up in time to figure out how to be married and why am I thinking I want one last shot at recklessness?

"That damn Tamoxifen!" I say, annoyed with the beads of sweat pooling under my hairline, at the small of my back, behind my knees, under the soft curve of my breast, and trickling down the center line that runs from the inner edge of my heart to the base of my groin. Had the cumulative effect of the drug finally kicked in? I sit up and peel off my boxers and my Bad Boy t-shirt, and feel awful that we have to waste time and energy discussing this problem I've caused. That it makes Mike feel inadequate. That I might cause even greater devastation. That all my layers have been stripped away. All the trying exhausted. And we're left with me lying sweaty and scarred and naked on the bed.

"Are you mad that I brought this on us?" I say and sputter, "I'm so sorry. . . . " I glance away and see him twenty years ago (we were just kids, what were we thinking? how could we know?) and me wanting him to see me as more perfect than I was or ever would be. And now I think how hard this marriage has been for him, how much happier he might have been with Rita or Laura New Hampshire or that blond-bobbed Episcopalian Dartmouth grad his mother had in mind for him, and I feel sad and sorry about that. And I worry that he sees too much of me, and I wonder if all these years the thought that I was *too much* for him was actually a mask for my *real* concern, that I wasn't enough. That I'm not.

"No," he says, cupping my face with both his hands and turning it toward him. "Are you kidding?" He brushes my hair out of my eyes and looks at me as openly and completely as anyone ever has, the way he looked at me when we first met, and says, "Not at all. I just wish I could have taken the hit for us."

He blinks a few times as if he might cry. But he doesn't cry, never cries the oceans of pent-up sadness in his eyes, enough to drown both of us in his sorrow, and makes me fall in love with his muffled vulnerability all over again.

"I wouldn't wish that on you," I say. "But I appreciate you saying that." And I crawl back under the comforter and think maybe we've evolved a tiny bit beyond his parents' marriage.

The mammogram waiting room is full of overly polite tension. All the women sit lined up on stiff padded chairs in matching cotton gowns and slippers, pretending to read magazines, waiting to be called for films and then waiting to either be called back for more films or told, "You can get dressed and go home," meaning you're okay.

It sort of reminds me of how it felt to audition for acting jobs. You'd wait in a room with all the other auditioners, studying one another and wondering who would get lucky. Although getting the callback for that was a good thing and here it's the opposite and the stakes are a teeny bit higher.

But I get called back several times and each time the other women nod at me empathetically while also trying to hide their relief that it isn't them. And in between the waiting, which goes on for a couple of hours, I catch myself thinking of myself in the past tense, *She was a mother, a wife, a failed novelist, an indifferent housekeeper and in spite of avoiding parabens and pesticides* . . . and watching the storm on the TV perched in the corner, record high winds and thunderstorms and flash flood warnings, and trying to figure out if that's a good sign or a bad sign. I never consider that it might be no sign at all.

Although I figure the more films I get, the more likely they're going to find something wrong, so I'm surprised, after eleven films, that I get the "Gail Baker? You can get dressed and go home." I jump up like a contestant on *Let's Make a Deal* and throw my arms around my technician and say, "Are you sure? Are you sure? Are you sure?"

She nods.

"Thank you. Thank you. Thank you."

It's two days before my forty-sixth birthday, and on the way home from the appointment it's still raining hard. But now the rain sounds like applause, and I keep thinking I should take a bow—I'm giddy with the feeling that I just got away with something I might not deserve. My mind races to all the things I can't wait to do and I ask Mike what he has planned for the birthday celebration.

"You said making plans made you feel superstitious," he says.

"And you listened to me?" I say. "I have six months to celebrate and I want a party and I want to go see Bonnie Raitt next week and I want to make the plane and room reservations for the half-marathon and I want to book a hotel room for the weekend we're driving Anna to college and maybe we should go to the city after that. We haven't been to New York in a while and I always like to go see our old apartment in The Village. . . . "

twenty

My Friend
Has an Affair
for Me

"The first time we did it on a sailboat leaning against the mast," Glenda, my old friend from college, says through the faint long-distance connection. "And a fishing boat floated up just as I was coming. What a rush! I feel like I'm twenty! I haven't felt this alive in years. I had no idea how numb I was . . . did I tell you . . . he's twenty-eight and huge!"

"Twenty-eight, huh?"

"I didn't realize how lacking Bob was in that department until . . . anyway, last night we snuck out at 3 A.M. and did it in the minivan and I came four times!"

"Four times, huh?" I say. "What are you going to do about Bob?"

"Screw Bob. He's in love with Tax Law. I can't remember the last time he looked at me, I mean *really* looked at me . . . I've been so . . . lonely." She pauses.

We both sigh.

"I'm doing this for 'us,'" she says. "You inspired me. Your scare reminded me that life is short and we have to seize pleasure wherever and whenever we can. I'm seizing our pleasure!"

"Wow. I guess I should thank you."

"No. No. I should thank you . . . do you think I'm a slut? Because I feel like maybe I'm a slut. All I want is sex sex sex sex sex. The more I have the more I want. I know Bob would think I was a slut if he found out and so would all my neighbors, not that I care what *they* think. But I *do* care what you think. . . . "

"No, I don't think you're a slut. I think you're gutsy and maybe a little crazy. I'm the slut."

"You? What does that mean?"

"It means I've mentally either made out or slept with more men than you can imagine. I'm a slut in my own mind."

She laughs. "That's hilarious. But you don't sleep with them all?"

"Not if they aren't good kissers . . . remember that little phone thing I had with the writer?"

"Did that involve phone sex?"

"No! No sex. No sex talk. But I imagined he was a great kisser."

"Talk about kissing, the kissing is phenomenal. Tender but also kind of commanding. He has these full lips and he's *very* good with his tongue in general and he's strong. He can lift me up and well the whole thing is so animalistic. Makes me realize we're all essentially animals. We screw, we eat, we reproduce and die. This is 'our' way of saying, Screw you, death."

"Are 'we' using protection?"

twenty-one

Running Through
Times Square

END OF AUGUST: I'm running through Central Park with my girlfriends in a sea of other runners, our legs like paddles powering the same crew boat. We move as one and it feels effortless. We circle the park and then we head down Seventh Avenue to 42nd Street, the neon billboards of Times Square flashing, live bands jamming, and colorful waves of runners bobbing just ahead, pulling us along in this tide of my fellow runners, my fellow human beings. *This is what it means to be alive. This is oneness with others. I could run forever and ever. . . .*

Until mile eleven, when I want to stop. Immediately. We're on the West Side Highway and it's too long and straight and it looks like the end is nowhere in sight. And my legs are too heavy. Each step feels like a mile and I'm reminded of how I felt after my mammogram. After my diagnosis. After my surgery. How hard it was to take the next step. To trust that taking the next step was possible, that it would actually move me forward. How I want to just sit down and stop. Now. Don't want to deal with anything this hard. Why did I agree to this? Why would I put myself through this?

My girlfriends surround me. They're both seasoned marathoners and racers and I can see that they can see that I've hit a wall.

"We're almost there," Martha says. "You can do it!"

I shake my head.

"Let's sing," Tina suggests.

They hook my elbows and we belt out, "I feel good," the rest of the way down that endless road, until we cross the finish line holding hands overhead in victory.

We're staying at the Tribeca Grand Hotel, which feels more like a nightclub than a hotel. Dim lights, dark walls, and the bar is always open, and there's an omnipresent techno beat that follows us everywhere, into the elevator and down the narrow hallways and into our room (unless we turn it off).

The morning we woke for the race at 5 A.M., there were sexy young thangs in slinky little things still sipping cocktails and making out on the couches from the night before. But I like the vibe because it doesn't remind me of family vacations, doesn't remind me of family at all, and now that the race is over, all we've been doing is eating and shopping and talking old boyfriends. It's like *Sex and the City*. Although no actual sex.

We sit on couches as vast as beds in half light in the hotel lounge sipping wine in wide-mouthed goblets, the techno beat throbbing as I say, "One time, on Mike and my sixteenth anniversary, I was getting us drinks at the bar and this thirty-something guy asked me, 'What was your most erotic sexual experience?' And I'm like, it's my sixteenth anniversary and my husband is right over there. And he shrugged and said, 'Okay I'll go first. Mine was on a beach in Brazil and there was a gorgeous woman and she didn't speak any English and she took my hand and placed it on my. . . . ' Mike slides up behind me then and he has no idea what we're talking about and I think, This may be my most erotic experience. . . . "

Martha and Tina laugh.

"That's pretty pathetic," Martha says. "One time, before I met Pete, I was at a club and I'd been flirting with this male ballet dancer all night and he said, 'Would you like to see me do a grande battement?' and he pulled me into this stairwell. . . . "

Our curly-haired waiter with the five o' clock shadow bends down to empty our spotless ashtray and glances at my girlfriends' cleavage-revealing shirts, the kind of shirt I would have worn before my surgery. Now I'm wearing a fitted tank top that scoops half an inch above the upper edge of my largest scar.

"Use your imagination," Martha says and the waiter grins as if she meant that comment for him.

"Wow, you topped me," I say and then I gulp, sort of choke on my wine when I lower my voice and say, "Not that I didn't have some mindless all-about-the-sex 'things' before I was married, but no grande battement, and the thing is . . . I don't feel very sexy since my surgery. I have four scars and one is really . . . noticeable and I can barely look at my chest in the mirror. Mike keeps saying, 'You're still beautiful' . . . but I feel like he doesn't mind it nearly as much as I do because. . . . "

"What?" Martha says.

"Never mind. It's stupid. . . . "

"No. No. Tell us."

"I feel like I'm . . . branded and that makes him think now I *couldn't* stray so that's why it doesn't bother him. . . . Is that crazy?"

"No. He's always been so jealous. I can see that. He *would* want you branded." Martha nods.

"It's not like I ever thought I'd *actually* have an affair, not that I haven't imagined it, but whenever Mike and I fought I always liked to think I was attractive enough that I *could* have an affair and now I'm so mad at myself. . . . "

"For what?" Tina asks.

I lean down and whisper even though it's loud and I don't know anyone here. "There was one guy . . . once . . . a writer . . . who I thought I *really* liked . . . you know about him, Martha."

"You mean that writer guy you couldn't stop talking to?"

I nod. "It was like we could finish each other's sentences. I felt like he just 'knew' me and 'got' me and he made me laugh and he liked my writing. . . . "

"What happened?" Tina says.

"Nothing. It was all on the phone and computer and I realized one of the things I found most attractive about him was the way he'd say his wife's name . . . with such respect and love . . . so I had a crush on a guy who was in love with his wife partly *because* he loved his wife. . . . "

"You *are* pathetic, aren't you?" Martha says.

"No, I think that's sweet," Tina says.

"But now, now I'm thinking why didn't I go meet him and pull him in a closet and make out and at least go to second base with him because . . . who would want me now?" My eyes land on my girlfriends' cleavage, on the lovely smooth slopes.

"Show us," Martha says.

"Show you what?"

"Your scar."

I gulp. When I undress, I cover my breasts even for myself, holding one hand over my flawed breast as I wrap my bra around my back, grasping the side with my elbow before snapping up fast and catching my flesh in the soft cups. But these are my girlfriends and they're the reason I'm here, the reason I had the motivation to train for this race when all I wanted to do was curl up in a ball and cry and try to figure out a way to rewind the clock. Martha dragged me out to run week after week even when I said I wasn't up for it and that helped me start to turn this crappy year around. We've run thirteen miles through Central Park and down 42nd Street and had three days of a 24/7 slumber party, three days in which I have fallen into such a comfortable routine that I imagine I am twenty-eight and never married or had kids, that I live in the city in a hotel nightclub, that I shop and eat and run and at night I sip wine to the techno beat . . . so I down the rest of my wine and scootch in closer to them and pull the neck of my tank top down. I inch my bra down and lean over the table and show them my scar.

We all stare at the pink raised flesh that cuts a thick, crooked slash across the upper portion of my breast.

No one says anything for a moment. I know it isn't pretty and I'm about to cover up when Martha says, "I think it's sexy."

Tina nods.

"Yeah, there's something really intriguing about a scar," Martha continues.

"I think if anything, it makes you sexier," Tina says.

"Makes you different."

"Flaws are hot."

I glance down and see where the virgin skin dead-ends into the wound. I wish it wasn't like that, wish I could undo the damage, but I can't. Can't change it, can't change what is, what happened. This is my body. The scar is me and I am the scar. And it's a symbol of what I've been through, a reminder that I've survived, and it makes me exactly who I am now. And if my girl-friends say that it makes me sexier, I'm going to try to hold on to that.

I'm teary eyed as I say, "Thanks guys, for saying that." I sit back up and let go of my bra and shirt and lean back into the sofa. "Maybe we should just stay in New York. Start over. We could get an apartment and find some fun jobs and share all the chores and have lots of casual lovers."

We all laugh as our waiter circles our table, emptying our unused ashtray again and insisting we order an-other round of drinks.

That night I fall asleep thinking, I want to be flirtier and sexier. More daring and interesting. I want to stop holding back. I want to experience more excitement and pleasure and joy because life is short . . . and I dream of my ballet dancer, my grande battement, and I think, Screw it. Why have I always said no no no? I say yes yes yes and we're doing it in the stairwell and he's strong and it feels amazing, but when I look up I see that the ballet dancer has his eyes closed and he's mas-saging his own sculpted torso.

I wake up in a flash and think: What have I done? What have I done? This guy doesn't love me. Mike loves me and . . . I love him in spite of all we've been through or maybe because of all we've been through and it occurs to me that staying wasn't cowardly. For me. Walking away, starting over, leaving all the unresolved messiness behind would have been easier. Staying has been the most difficult and complicated piece of my life, my PhD, the dissertation I may never complete.

Back in Madison, I call Dawn and we walk and she tells me all her good news. That her clinical trial is going even better than expected. That people have been so kind and generous to her. That she's tolerating the chemo. Hasn't lost too much hair. That she's taken up meditation and has been studying Buddhism, getting massages, juicing, taking the best care of herself ever . . . and the only thing really bothering her is that Bush is still in office. And I leave her thinking, She's going to survive.

twenty-two

Letting Go

THE WEEK BEFORE we take Anna to college is all about getting her ready to go. We shop for dorm-room stuff, comforters and rugs and posters, and sort through her room to decide what to take and what to leave. She's bringing her favorite teddy bear and the stuffed moon-and-stars baby mobile and leaving her collection of Beanie Babies and Gel Roll pens.

I remember reading that when Sylvia Plath was home with her two little children, she just wanted to get everything done, all the chores, all the endless tasks, so she wouldn't have to *do* them anymore. And while that was just shortly before she killed herself and was an illustration of her frustration and inability to cope, I understood how she felt. There were plenty of times I felt that way. Plenty of times the day moved so slowly I felt like I was walking through pond sludge. And I wondered why I was being tortured with endless drudgery turning my brain to mush . . . but now I want the days to expand. Elongate.

I want sitting cross-legged on Anna's bedroom floor, elbow to knee, sorting through books and mementoes to go on forever.

"What about *Goodnight Moon?*" Anna says, fingering the nearly shredded book.

"That was your favorite," I say. "'Goodnight room. Goodnight moon.'"

"'Goodnight cow jumping over the moon,'" she chimes in and smiles and tosses it in the Things To Take box, reminding me how much we both loved that book.

I'd never been one of those Goo-Goo Baby Women. Never babysat much as a teenager. Never fussed over other people's babies. In fact, I hadn't pictured marriage or babies until I met Mike. Then a couple of years after that, when I suddenly started dreaming and thinking about babies obsessively, the next thing I knew I was in the hospital amazed I'd pushed a baby into the world. She was crying and the nurse handed her to me and the exquisite heft of her warm, pillowy body against mine was so much more substantial, more rewarding than anything I'd ever expected.

Those little fingers—who knew they'd be the most perfect fingers in the world? And all ten! With teeny tiny nails and a fierce grip. She took a little breath and it sent a shiver through me and I thought, So this is love, love in its purest form, love based on biology and evolution and the feel of her buttery forearm. This is the reason I was put on earth. To hold my baby in my arms, to slow my breath to the rhythm of her breath. She gurgled! I couldn't believe it. What a beautiful sound. The most beautiful sound I'd ever heard. She breathed and all I wanted to do was watch her breathe again, marvel in the tenderness of her skin, gaze into her already wise eyes. I couldn't believe that I'd created a human being who could gurgle. Gurgle and breathe. Gurgle and breathe. Perhaps that was my finest moment of motherhood. . . .

"Mom? Mom? Do you think I should take my old baby doll?" Anna says, nodding at the bald-headed baby doll in her arms.

"Do you want to?" I ask.

She nods, a little sheepishly.

"Absolutely," I say and she plops it in the box on top of *Goodnight Moon* and we keep sorting.

•   •   •

Time keeps hurtling forward, the drawers and closets emptying, the suitcases and boxes overflowing, and before I know it we've reached the end of the week. We've rented a U-Haul and the plan is for Mike and Anna to drive out to New York with the stuff and for me to fly out with Maddy and Alex a few days later.

It's a long drive for Anna and Mike, a long time for them to be alone together, and they both call me from their cell phones to complain the other one isn't saying anything (they share that British trait of letting the other person carry the conversation), which works when they are with chatty people (like Maddy and Alex and me) around to fill in the quiet space but makes both of them overly self-conscious of the silence when they're alone.

Mike loves her (loves all the kids) and he's slowly grown into the kind of dad I wish I'd had, the kind who would do anything for her (and incidentally wouldn't leave their mother), who is more than willing and happy to pack up and drive her to college even though he has such a hard time conversing with her (and I know that's discomfiting for him).

I feel the tension through the phone and wish I had more time to work on their relationship, but I tell them they have to work it out. Then I hang up the phone and try not to worry about it the rest of the day.

The morning of our flight, Mike calls and says there was an aborted terrorist attack in England, explosives hidden in hand luggage and the terrorist alert has been increased to the highest level. They're not letting people carry on any makeup or toiletries.

"That's crazy," I say, thinking he must be exaggerating. "And we're running late for our flight." I hang up the phone.

But he's right. The airport is swarming with security and long lines and signs about the high alert and all the things you can't bring on the flight, and I wonder whether it's wise to fly with Maddy and Alex on such a risky day.

I call Mike and say, "I don't know if we should get on the flight or not. Maybe we should drive instead."

"It's a long drive. It's okay. Don't come. We can handle it without you."

I hear Anna in the background, saying, "Give me the phone. Now. Give it to me." There's the sound of shuffling and then to me she says, "Don't listen to him. You have to come. Get on the plane. We haven't said goodbye."

We file into the long security line and give up our toiletries (including some very expensive organic paraben-free lotion I just bought because I gave up on making that fresh stuff every couple of days), and I tell the kids it will be fine and pray I'm not making a foolish choice just so Anna and I can say goodbye and we board the plane.

•   •   •

The Bard college campus is an eclectic hodgepodge of architecturally disparate buildings from gothic to cottagy to ultra-modern dotting a hilly stretch of land edged by the Hudson river and a view of the Catskill mountains in the distance.

"This is spectacular!" I say, all the while thinking about how different it was for me when I went off to college. My older brother Daniel had been at Simon's Rock and was transferring and my dad called me up one day and said, "Would you like to go to college?" I was sixteen and I couldn't wait to get away from the confusion of moving back and forth between my parents' houses, switching schools, feeling like I was a burden and an outsider wherever I landed, so I said, "Yes!" And the next thing I knew I was on a train to Great Barrington, Massachusetts. Alone. With my trunk. And a little cash. So I'm not totally clear how to do this taking-the-daughter-to-college thing.

"Will you get a look at that performing arts center?" I say in my overly eager voice.

We follow the signs to Keen North, drive up a gravel path. "The dorm is lovely!" I exclaim. It's a plain clapboard building with a tacked-on front porch. "And all the students look so smart!" I point to two students locking up their bikes.

The kids and Mike look at me as if I've lost it. "They do," I say, nodding my head, as Mike pulls the U-Haul up as close as we're able.

We meet Anna's roommate and her parents on our way into the dorm. They seem nice, a little older, tell us this is their youngest, they've been here for hours already, done this before, ask, "Do you want to go in on a refrigerator?"

We nod and then we begin the long impossible-looking job of unpacking the U-Haul and car. The trips back and forth take hours but there is something relaxing in the repetitive task of lifting and carrying and unloading. I guess this is what is meant by the Buddhist saying: "Before enlightenment, chop wood and haul water. After enlightenment, chop wood and haul water." At some point it seems as if the stuff isn't going to fit in her small room but we bring it in anyway. Unload and stack. Chop and haul.

The Other Mother seems to be working off a master list and shaking her head at all the inadequacies of the room, as I lean the license plate from our last car in Vermont on Anna's windowsill and tack up James Dean.

The Other Mother says they need more shelving and hooks and bed risers and the refrigerator. Mike and Alex are already on their way to Target and the hardware store for light bulbs and extension cords and Mike offers to get the refrigerator for the girls.

I stay back with Anna and Maddy and while Anna works on arranging the closet, and Maddy checks her Facebook on the computer, I put clothes away in the bureau. The Other Mother is putting clothes away, too. Only I notice she's doing it a lot more carefully than I am. She's taking each pair of underwear and smoothing it out with the palm of her hand and then rolling it into a neat cylinder. I reach for Anna's underwear that I've shoved in the top drawer and I start smoothing and rolling, smoothing and rolling. Tucking each pair into the drawer, thinking I should color coordinate at the same time, keep all the like colors together. . . .

Anna clears her throat and I look up as she mouths, "What are you doing?"

"Putting your underwear away?" I say.

She shakes her head, walks over, and whispers, "You have *never* folded my underwear and I don't want you to start now."

Maddy glances up from the computer screen and chuckles. I'm sure the Other Mother has heard this and I'm a little embarrassed but I close the drawer and work on finding a place for Marilyn Monroe.

By late afternoon, we've made several trips to the health food store to stock up on food and the general store to stock up on detergent and we've been to the bookstore for books and school supplies. We heard that Jessica Lange's and Sam Shepard's son and Francis Ford Coppola's granddaughter are also freshmen, so we spend a little time star-stalking the campus, but soon tire of not finding them and realize they're probably keeping a low profile because of people like me. Then we head back to

Anna's room and look for more things we need to do. But the bed is made, the posters are hung, the shelves are up, and parents are starting to say goodbye.

Except for the Other Mother, who has crawled (for the third time) underneath her daughter's bed, trying to flatten out the carpet a little more? Or is she after a dust ball? We all watch the mother's legs dangle and flop and I think, Okay she wins. She's the better mother. There's no contest. She folds underwear and crawls under beds.

Just when I'm thinking maybe there is something under Anna's bed I need to do, her daughter turns to me and says, "I'm having a *Wizard of Oz* flashback here."

We all bite our lips and try not to grin and the father rolls his eyes and says, to his wife's shoes, "That's enough, dear. Time to go."

Then before I know it, we're all standing in the quad. Anna and I look at each other and we both reach out, our chests pressing together. We're cheek to cheek and she's four and we're in the cloakroom of her nursery school and the other mothers say a quick goodbye, but when we hug, Anna whispers in my ear, "Don't ever let go until I'm ready." And then she's seventeen, a high school senior on stage for her final chorus concert this past spring, and I see her first nursery school concert, how when they got to the part when the kids were supposed to jingle their bells, she didn't have a bell and she dissolved into tears and so did I.

But now she sings with the self-possession of the re-markable young woman she's grown into. She doesn't need a jingle bell, doesn't need me worrying whether she has one. And as I stand here in the quad I feel the rush of all the years passing in this moment. I didn't mean to rush it. I didn't mean to ever feel frustrated and bored, to want to get everything done, to ever think, When she finally grows up I'll get my life back, because it isn't true. She was and is my life and *I'm* not ready to let go . . . and we're both crying now, our bod-ies trembling as she whispers, "It's okay, Mom. We're both going to be okay."

Back in Madison, I walk through Anna's room, feeling the hollowness of the space without her essence. I pick up things she left behind, the frilly pink basket full of headbands and butterfly clips, fluff the pillows on her bed, straighten row after row of picture books, and imagine her in her dorm room, meeting new people, starting classes on Monday, the whole world opening up to her and think, It's time for me to stop dicking around and get back to work.

I e-mail my agent and tell her while I'm very appre-ciative of all the work she has done on my behalf, I think it's time for us to part ways. She e-mails me back and says, while she's sorry to see us part, she under-stands. And I'm free. Free to do whatever I want with my writing life.

Which is a little scary because I'm not sure what to do with it. Still, I march myself out to my hut (telling myself it isn't a mausoleum, it's a room of my own and what I always wanted and an utter waste not to use it) and I spend the next few days setting it up.

There's already an old desk and chair and bookshelf that Mike moved in months ago. But I haul out things that I love: my Audrey Hepburn *Breakfast at Tiffany's* and *We Can Do It* posters. My postcards, including Andy Warhol's "The world fascinates me," my Marilyn Monroes, my assorted Leonardo da Vinci sketches, my favorite *New Yorker* cartoons and random quotes I love like "Well-behaved women rarely make history" and Emily Dickinson's "Dwell in possibility," some old floral hatboxes I bought at an estate sale, an enormous dictionary and thesaurus, my beaten-up copies of *Anna Karenina* and *The Great Gatsby,* my ribbons and bibs from my road races, my Grandmother Elsie's old engraved sugar holder (the only thing of hers I have), which I fill with my favorite pens, a beeswax candle, a decoupaged box of Michelangelo's hands from the Sistine Chapel (that my friend Allison bought me when we were roommates in The Village), and a little brass Indian lady (given to me by our Indian neighbors in New Hampshire many years ago) that represents success.

And even though I'm not a very religious or ritualistic person, when I'm done I kneel down and light the candle and bow forward and plant my hands firmly on the earth and thank God for my health and the health of Anna and Maddy and Alex and Mike, and then I offer my day to Dawn and her children and others who are suffering more than I am.

I ask God, whomever he, she, it may be, to fill me full of love, compassion, patience, hope, trust, balance, honor, endurance, and humility and I ask for the wisdom and courage and passion to be the most amazing me and I say to myself, "I believe in your infinite wisdom and I am open to whatever you may have to teach me and please point me in the direction of my dreams and also, please bring me the mojo."

Then I cup my breasts and say, "I am strong, I am healthy, I am healed," and I do a spinal twist on both sides and a head stand for a count of thirty and a downward-facing dog and a backbend and hang forward and slowly roll up and reach my arms overhead and ask for the mojo again. And then I thank Anna for inspiring me to get my shit together, and I ask for some mojo for her and then sit down and write.

I do this same exact thing over the course of several days and I end up writing an essay based on my recovery journals. I lay it all out, holding nothing back, the anger, the fears, the wild and contradictory thoughts that ran through my head and I'm weeping as I title it *Cancer Is a Bitch.*

I show it to Mike, who shakes as he reads it and says, "Wow, that's . . . intense."

"I think it might be the best thing I've ever written."

"What about your novels?"

I shrug and then I point down and tap the pages. "This is the real deal. This is me on the page. Well, and a little you, although you notice I refer to you as 'my husband.'"

He nods.

"You're okay with this, right?"

He nods again. "Sure, it's fine. You do what you have to do."

And I think how strange, considering how resistant he was to talking about our lives with a therapist, that he's okay with me sharing our lives with the world. And what about me not wanting the responsibility of being "The Woman Who Had Breast Cancer"? What am I thinking? Maybe we're both thinking this will end up in a box just like the novels and no one will read it.

I send it to a few writer friends for feedback anyway. One who asks me, "Who is your intended market?"

"I'm not sure," I write back. "What do you think?"

"I think you might want to tone it down . . . I wouldn't call it *Cancer Is a Bitch*. It sounds a little . . . bitchy. Otherwise, it's amazing."

I trust this writer and I know she's only telling me this to help me get it published. And then I think, Screw it. Cancer *is* a bitch!

One day soon after that, I read that *Literary Mama* is looking for columnists and on an absolute whim, I chop up the essay into shorter pieces and I pitch them the idea of it as a column and they invite me to send them a few rough samples. When they offer me a monthly column, "Bare-breasted Mama," swearing and all, I love and respect, absolutely adore them for that, even as I wonder why I'm choosing to bare myself this way.

twenty-three

Mother Writes
a Letter to Oprah

DEAR OPRAH,

When I watch you on television and read *O*, I feel like I am spending time with a best friend. We are so similar, you and I; despite antithetical backgrounds and pathways, our struggles, aspirations, and values are the same. I grew up white, rich, and abused in the mid-west. You grew up black, poor and abused in the south. We were both little girls whose spirit, hope and self identity were so critically challenged, by the physical and emotional pain we sustained, and by the "secrets" we hid inside out of fear and protection of our abusers, it's amazing we turned out as we did. Where I am most like you, Oprah, is in utilizing my personal experience of suffering, to do what I can to allevi-

ate suffering in others. I am a 70 year old occupational therapist, who works in a clinic, and travels around the country
teaching occupational and physical therapists how to treat
patients with Parkinson's disease. I wanted you to know something about me before I tell you why I am writing this letter to
you.

My daughter, Gail, is a breast cancer survivor. A busy
mother of 3, runner, part-time Yoga instructor, and writer, she
refused to succumb to the physical and emotional wounds of
breast cancer. Rather than be intimidated by this ultimate enemy of all women, she began a literary column called "Bare-
breasted Mama," where she lays open her fear, her pain, her
shock at being diagnosed with cancer. Six weeks after her surgery, she was running again, preparing for a half-marathon.
Oprah, Gail would make a riveting guest on your show. She is
funny and intelligent, and courageous.

"Did you get the letter?" my mother, who has been
reading my column online, asks me on the phone. "Was
it six weeks after surgery you were running? I was going
to put in how cute you are but I thought that was
overkill. I'm sure we'll hear soon. Don't you love how I
started it out with that personal connection? That is
going to get her. She's going to feel that and want both
of us on the program. I'm just so proud of you and that
'Bare-breasted Mama' thing. It's so bold. A little
raunchy even." She laughs. "I didn't know you had such
a powerful voice." She giggles. "Oh honey, you're so tal-
ented. And I went to your website and I've been reading everything you've written. I can't stop. It's all so
riveting! That story about the mother who has to waitress after her husband leaves her for a younger woman

and she has a nervous breakdown? I love it. But did my legs actually squish-squish together in my support hose? Could you make her legs just a little thinner?"

My mother's flattery and attention can pull me in and suck me under with more power and finesse than a tidal wave, making me forget how quickly she can yank it away. I know that, yet I can't help but enjoy her praise, a little, even though I don't trust it entirely. But I hang up the phone believing her words, imagining she always praised me that way.

Not a week later my Aunt Arlene, who thinks I've lost my breasts and is so hard of hearing she doesn't hear me when I say I haven't, calls and launches into a story about some man she knows who picked up a very attractive forty-something woman in a bar and took her to a motel and she undressed and he said she had the most perfect body he'd ever seen and the woman started laughing and told him she'd had a bilateral mastectomy and reconstruction. "And he lost his erection," my aunt says. "This is a man who screws anything! I heard they can tuck your tummy at the same time. Your cousin Morty knows a Chinese herbalist who specializes in cancer victims who aren't responding to treatment. I'm sorry you're the only one in the family who's ever *had* cancer." And then we're disconnected.

"What did you tell Arlene?" I try not to scream at my mother as I open the refrigerator and jiggle the OJ and milk containers, toss old leftovers into the sink.

"Remember, your negativity isn't healthy," she says. "I told her I've been going through a rough time because my lovely Gail was stricken with cancer."

"Did you tell her that I still have my breasts? That they got it all out? That it was noninvasive and I had a good checkup in July?"

"You know she's hard of hearing. She doesn't listen anyway. It's amazing she wasn't afraid to call you. She thinks cancer is contagious."

"I'm hanging up," I say. "I can't have this conversation." For one thing, I need to go to the grocery store, I think.

"Oh, honey. I don't want this to get in the way of our relationship. I value our connection. You know my family's screwy and all their money did nothing, *nothing* for me. You know Mother married Daddy for money and she was the most self-absorbed human being on earth and she didn't want me. Getting her hair done was more important than me. She told me she'd never love me like she loved the others, especially Ronnie who was her favorite. . . . "

I've heard this story a million times about Grandmother Elsie, who I always secretly liked, even though my mother didn't, because she was so different from Gramma Rosie. Slim and elegant and fashionable, she always wore fitted camel-colored slacks and cashmere sweaters and silk scarves and she was unusually restrained for a Jewish Grandmother. She always chewed Wrigley Spearmint gum and brought us presents from fancy stores wrapped in tissue paper and she smelled like Chanel No. 5. And, it was true, she favored her oldest son, Ronnie. Gave him more of everything, more money and love and attention and in a sad twist, his daughter, my cousin Shelly, who was my age, died the day of my Grandmother Elsie's funeral. In fact, we were all milling about in the lobby of the temple just before the service when one of Shelly's brothers came in to announce that they'd found Shelly dead in a grocery store parking lot. She lived like a rock star and died like a homeless woman.

"Where is this going, Mom?" I ask now.

Maddy and Alex are coming in the house now from school and both mouthing, "Who are you talking to?"

"My mother," I mouth back, and they set their books down at the dining room table and I close the refrigerator door and find a pad and make a list. Fruit, milk, eggs, yogurt, something EASY for dinner.

"I don't want to pass this legacy down," my mother is saying. "I've come to peace with my own mother and the ways she hurt me and I want us to . . . well, I've been meaning to tell you . . . I'm, I'm . . . sorry. I screwed up, with you and Daniel and the other kids. I didn't know how to be a mother. I was too immature. And . . . and I want to know if you can forgive me."

I'm floored by this confession, this remarkably lucid sense of self-awareness, followed by a genuine apology, no less. I am about to tell her that I *do* forgive her and that I understand how hard it was for her. But before I can speak, she says, "Now I need you to give me something. I need you to tell me that I gave you intelligence and passion and a terrific sense of humor and your brilliant ironic outlook. I mean, look at you. Look at the woman you've grown into. Trust me, you wouldn't be who you are if I'd been like Susie Day's mother."

Susie Day, daughter of the parents who lit up when she walked into a room and loved her unconditionally.

"Although I *did* have my super-mom moments," she's still saying. "Remember when I used to sew all your clothes? And made all those fun birthday parties in the backyard and how about those tissue-paper flowers in your favorite shocking pink . . . and remember when you came back to Toledo and we went to college together?"

Of course I remember. After Daniel's first nervous breakdown, I left Simon's Rock because I was confused and felt guilty about being away from home so I moved back to Toledo and spent very little time with Daniel because he . . . scared me. . . . He was different doped up on meds, had a sort of zombie quality, as if he'd entered another realm that I didn't know how to reach, and when I saw him I was convinced it was just a matter of time before I *became* him. So I got busy, got a job selling men's clothing, and a cheap apartment across from the notorious drug-selling park and after six months of that, I went back to finish up my degree at the University of Toledo, where my mother was finishing up a master's in philosophy.

That year we hung out, meeting for lunch in the faculty lounge and writing papers together at her apartment. She was so focused and thorough and brilliant, the darling of the Philosophy Department, even revered in the English Department, where I lived in her shadow. And I learned about passion and determination, about how to take an idea and follow it through to the very end and then back again a few more times.

In some ways, that year felt like it made up for the years of neglect—until I left for New York City and she dumped me for her second husband, the octogenarian self-made millionaire, whom she divorced in an ugly battle a few years later.

"We had so much fun, remember how we always shared the Greek salad light on the feta in the faculty lounge? And I introduced you to the existentialists and Plato," she's saying now.

Now I feel sick, the ground swelling, the list receding, my hands trembling. This is the tidal wave and it reminds me too much of the conversation with my dad a few years back when I tried to tell him how I felt about him leaving us, and he twisted the whole thing back to him. But I don't give her what she's asking me for. I can't.

Instead, I say, "Hold on." Then I walk with the phone into the living room so my kids can't hear me. "You're asking me to forgive you but you also want me to tell you how wonderful and smart you were? What a good influence? I don't want to play that game. And to be honest with you, you abandoning me, abandoning us, traumatized me so much that I've spent most of my adult life feeling guilty for having survived my childhood and so determined not to abandon my own children that I forgot about me." And I think, ironically, I may end up abandoning my children anyway.

"Oh, honey. No, you misunderstand me. I didn't mean that. I know I was a screwup. I wasn't worthy of you. . . . I had no right thinking I could raise children. I'm sorry. Really, I am . . . and I'm sorry I said that. And I want you to know that I've apologized to Daniel. I pray to him all the time and tell him how sorry I am . . . so I don't want you to worry about that."

I feel tears pooling behind my eyes because, damn it, I'm still not over Daniel. When would be a good time to get over this? Now would be a good time. Now. But just hearing his name slays me. Fills my head with unanswered questions: What was in the note? Was it schizophrenia or despair? Or both? Or neither? Bad family? Bad meds? Bad therapy? Bad genes?

And why didn't I know? Why didn't I *do* something? Say something? Stop him? Why wasn't I there? Why did I move to New York thinking that by leaving I could actually escape? And what would the answers do now? But I'm also tearing up because . . . this is different from other conversations we've had, different from the conversation I tried to have with my dad. My mother is actually saying some things I've wanted to hear her say for years.

Still, I'm not ready to tell her how much it makes my heart ache, not ready to let her hear me cry, so I let the waves of sadness wash over me before I say, "Thanks, Mom, I appreciate you saying that and it's true you did give me all those things, the intellect and wit and curiosity and passion and I draw on that a lot . . . and as a woman I get the bind you were in. . . . I get it. I've felt it. But as your daughter, you see, I *was* part of the bind and that's why I can't say it was okay you couldn't deal with my needs. The truth is, a kid doesn't necessarily need an interesting mother. A kid needs her Mom home with dinner or at least a plan for dinner and asking her if she has homework and how was her day and don't stay out too late. That's what was missing for me, for us, the boring old regular stuff . . . so while I do forgive you, I can't take away your pain of regret and I don't think that's my job. . . . " I'm a little nervous about saying all that, but what's the point of holding back now?

I'm surprised when she doesn't get angry. When she says, "You're right. I failed you as a mother and a woman but the point is . . . I love and admire everything about you and I miss you. Miss us."

I nod and I'm tearing up again. What a sap I am. When will I ever stop longing for that closeness, for the mother she *could* be?

"And . . . you're doing it all just right," she continues. "Mothering. The writing. Your marriage."

"That's not true," I say. "I'm not doing it all just right and don't idealize my life. I have my own struggles with the same issues. I think most women do. And I have my own regrets . . . and to be perfectly honest sometimes the hurt is still raw. . . . " The tears rise up again, but I swallow them back and manage to whisper, "Just like you with your own mother?"

"Look, my mother was horrid. Horrid. There are things I haven't even told you. . . . But what I learned from Mother Mary was that my mother was perfect for me because I wouldn't be the woman I am without having gone through what I did and I think that's true for you, too."

I'm not sure how Mother Mary got into the conversation but I say, "You're right."

"And I'm, I'm . . . your biggest fan," she says. "I'm not kidding you. You're writing the best damn prose today and you know how well-read I am—"

"Okay Mom, enough with the flattery. . . . " Although I do like it that she finally realizes I am capable of doing something in addition to mothering.

"You think I'm kidding? I'm not kidding and when I give my talks on Parkinson's, I always tell a little story about you. How brave you are. What an inspiration to me."

"Well, thank you," I say. "I'm flattered."

"And I sent the letter to Oprah and I'm sure we're going to hear soon," she says. "Oh, and I'm getting baptized next month," she says. "Did I tell you that?"

"With a white frilly gown and everything?"

"No, probably not a gown." She giggles. "But Jesus and Father Frank inspired me to grow as a person. Can't you tell?"

I'm not sure it's Father Frank or Jesus who has made a difference but I have to admit there is a difference. And while I want to get over all this and trust her fully, I don't. I can't. Not fully. Not yet. But maybe a little more than before.

As soon as I hang up, I walk back into the dining room where the kids are hunched over their papers and books strewn across the table and say, "I'm sorry."

"For what?" Maddy asks.

"For all the mistakes I've made and will continue making." I wave my hands overhead and all around.

They study me and then exchange looks with each other.

"Can you forgive me?" I ask.

"Maybe," Alex says. "If you make us some home-made cookies."

"Cookies? Right now?" I like to cook but I hate making cookies. "Not today. I have a column draft due tomorrow. But I'll put some on a plate for you."

twenty-four

The Purple Bra

FROM THE TIME my parents divorced, the holidays were always the starkest reminder of all that wasn't right in my family. The utter disregard for and extinction of our past, the incineration of our traditions and all that defined us a family unit, all that made us feel we deserved to belong to something that would endure.

The first couple of years after the divorce, my mother spent the holidays curled up on the couch. Later, when she got a job waitressing at The Big Boy (before she finally went back to school), she worked the holidays because they paid time and a half. My dad and stepmother would have us over at their new house, done up in my stepmother's ultra-modern style; all bold colors and sensually shaped sofas and flashy throw pillows and see-through table tops and long-haired rugs and aggressively splashy oil paintings, many she had painted. It wasn't just the décor. All of it was weird and unfamiliar. The smells, the conversation, the foods, especially the foods. My mother in her better-mother days was a fabulous cook. No matter what she made it was delicious (she had a slew of special dishes we all loved but she could make even a plate of cut fruit irresistible).

But my stepmother? What was she? Not a girl, but not quite a woman, and what did I expect her to be to me? She fascinated and frightened me with her clingy outfits and kittenish voice, her hypnotic hold on my dad and her utter lack of effort to win us over. Maybe I envied her cool, her entitlement. She was twenty-eight. How could I blame her for not knowing how or what to cook?

Even the packaged stuff she bought was weird. Like the "other" brand of graham crackers. And most of our meals with them were out at restaurants or takeout or frozen dinners. But on Thanksgiving she'd make this sweet potato casserole with marshmallows that we all hated, and my dad would always make a big fuss about how wonderful it was (probably because she never cooked otherwise), and then insist we all have some. For years I blamed that sweet potato casserole for ruining Thanksgiving. Really, it was because, while her extended family tried to be nice, they treated us like very distant cousins they didn't want to have to acknowledge.

And Christmas—which wasn't really Christmas for us, since we were Jewish, although we weren't all that religious about Hanukah even before the divorce, other than lighting the candles—turned into Let's-Give-the-Kids-a-Pile-of-Unwrapped-Presents Day. I don't know why the fact that they never wrapped the presents bugged me so much, but it did.

And my stepmother always picked me out an "outfit," which, because I was chubby, never fit right, and she'd *insist* I try it on. Then we'd all see how bad I looked in it and I'd end up returning it after the holidays and buying jeans on sale and pocketing the rest of the money.

And we'd go out to a Chinese restaurant and then I'd head over to my friend Stacey's where there was always a giant, perfectly symmetrical, fake tree, meticulously decorated (they'd actually measure the space between the color-coordinated balls) with matching ribbons and just the right amount of tinsel and tons of presents that looked professionally wrapped and tied up with bows and bells and other tasteful doodads. And there was a big ham and turkey and lots of eggnog and the parents getting so drunk that there'd be a huge family fight and the kids would have to break it up and put the parents to bed. Then they'd have their own party . . . and I'd come home stoned (I *did* smoke a little pot back then), to find my mother just home, exhausted from a long day of waitressing, and she'd tell me that she thought holidays were overrated and just another way for a capitalist society to force people into spending too much money.

And then she'd say once she got her feet on the ground we'd start celebrating. Maybe we should go somewhere warm, an island or something. And I'd tell her not to worry, that I thought the holidays were overrated and sitting with her on her mattress on the floor under her small metal energy pyramid suspended overhead, sipping herbal tea and talking, was way better than what most people did.

Then I met Mike's family, who, I thought, did Christmas just right. They cut down their tree from the Christmas tree farm and wrapped up lots of thoughtful gifts. They always threw a neighborhood party full of good cheer.

And after they got over the fact that their son was marrying a Jew, they got a kick out of my not having grown up with a real Christmas, and they made an even bigger deal out of it *for* me—and they loved how much I loved it. When our children were born it was even better—so much fun at Grammy and Grampa's house!—with lots of toys and sweets and Santa, until Mike's sister couldn't get pregnant. Finally she did, and a few short years later her oldest was diagnosed with autism—and because they were grieving and felt it was unfair (and it *was* and *is* unfair)—I think they found it too painful to deal with our healthy children. So, we stopped spending holidays with Mike's family.

After that we made our own holiday rituals, involving stockings and a tree cut down from the tree farm and latkes and Hanukah candles and *wrapped* presents for both holidays. When we moved to the Midwest, we started getting together with my sister and brother for Thanksgiving, alternating houses.

This was especially great for all the cousins, who bonded immediately and loved spending time together as we all got to know one another again. My brother and I falling right back into our old sarcastic banter, my sister and I sharing clothes and mothering stories and filling one another in on the years we'd lost. This went on joyfully for several years, until the year Mike and I had finally crawled out of debt and we were planning a trip to Paris, where my sister had been many times because her husband was from France and they'd always traveled, and I felt a shift in our relationship.

While she and her husband had always been financially comfortable (he's a polymer scientist who works for P&G and descended from French dry-cleaning moguls and she teaches French and dance), once we paid off our debt we were slightly more comfortable than them. Not that I cared. It was just that I felt that my sister liked me better when we were struggling, when she would call me from Europe and suggest we meet them for a fun weekend and I'd have to say, "Are you kidding? Mike has no time off and I just charged this week's groceries on the credit card."

Or maybe going even further back to our childhood when she was the dancer, the cutey, the honor roll student and I was floundering, the one who could never please, the one least likely to succeed. Maybe *that* was the relationship she was most comfortable with. I'm not sure. All I know is the Thanksgiving following our trip to Paris, we sat in my sister's kitchen sipping wine and my brother, always a bit of a provocateur, turned to my husband and said, "Hey, you wanna go test-drive a Jaguar?"

I kicked him under the table but it was too late. My sister's face tightened and the next year she called to say they were going skiing over Thanksgiving and that being with me made her feel worse about herself. I was shocked and hurt. Devastated. Still am.

Not to mention a little pissed at my brother, although he still claims it was the Paris trip that did it. I called her many times after that, telling her we had no interest in Jaguars and asking her what I had done to make her not want to see me. Was it something I said? Because I was sorry. And she just kept saying, "It isn't you. It's me." And while we still get together with my brother and his family for Thanksgiving, I haven't seen her since.

This is the oversized beat-up duffle bag I've dragged into the marriage, the one I'm always trying to kick away when, starting around mid-November and all the way through January, I walk around with an achy pit in my stomach, trying hard to feel festive but mostly feeling blue.

This year we fly to my brother's house in Atlanta even though Mike has to work the Friday after Thanksgiving and Anna has to fly in from New York and then fly back with us to Madison the next day and then back to college two days after that. The whole thing is rushed and complicated and exhausting and the kids are not thrilled about it, but since it's the only extended-family thing we do, Mike and I insist.

My sister-in-law makes a Southern low-carb Thanksgiving meal, since she's from Texas and my brother is low-carb again. Except for the cranberry sauce and biscuits she makes every year, and my kids love, it includes mostly unfamiliar foods: collard greens and pies made with the sweetener stevia; a turkey basted in a bag with soy sauce. And we eat outside under the hot Georgian sun and even though it's great to be together, I can tell the kids don't think it feels like Thanksgiving and of course this makes me think of my stepmother's sweet potato casserole.

As soon as we're on the plane home, Anna tells me one of the things she missed most about home was the food and she wonders if we can cook our own Thanksgiving and also all the foods she's been dreaming about.

So we spend the weekend cooking. In addition to turkey and stuffing and squash and mashed potatoes, I make Anna's favorite spanikopita and Turkish salad and grilled salmon marinated in orange juice and fresh ginger and garlic and rubbed with turmeric-infused olive oil and that chunky apple walnut cake with the warm Calvados sauce.

And all we do is eat and talk and talk and eat and eat and talk. And, at least for the weekend, I put most of my food anxieties aside and enjoy the pleasure of sharing food with people I love and I'm pretty sure it's the best Thanksgiving we've ever had.

Soon it's Hanukah and Christmas, which we wrap into one Big Holiday with endless presents and candle lighting and latkes (which Alex *loves* and helps me make) and another turkey and a trip to the Christmas store for a huge wood-carved Santa. The kids ask me why on earth I bought the Santa when none of them believes in Santa anymore and I'm Jewish. I don't have a good answer but I find myself smiling as I unwrap it and place it on top of the piano.

On New Year's Eve, Mike and I stop in at my friend Tina's, where, last year, I'd joked about not wanting to grow older. I tell Tina I take it back; I'm thrilled to be growing older. She laughs and we toast and hug. Then we head over to my wise friend Rachel's party full of her inimitable spirit and warmth, her radiant smile and intuitive charm, and her kitchen overflowing with salads, dips, nuts, salmon, sweets, and plenty of organic fruits and veggies (I know she picked them out with me in mind). A lot of our friends are there, including Dawn Myers, who tells all of us that her treatment has been so successful that they can't detect any cancer on the PET scan.

She's cured! She's cured! I'm so happy I'm practically shaking. "It's a miracle," I say.

Dawn laughs. "I don't believe in miracles," she says. "You know I'm an atheist."

"Birth is a miracle," someone says.

"What about the parting of the sea?" another person says.

"Birth is a biological phenomenon," Dawn says. "And the parting of the sea?" She shrugs and chuckles.

And even though I *do* believe in miracles, I love it that even after all she's been through this year, she's still so feisty, so clear in her convictions. So *her*.

"Have I shown you this?" Dawn flashes me her countdown-for-Bush key chain. Only 751 more days until the end.

I laugh. "That's hopeful," I say. She hasn't missed a beat.

Then everybody's talking Bush and the war and more religion and meditation (which Dawn *does* believe in now) and movies and music and global warming and gay marriage and Hillary Clinton and where did Rachel get the recipe for that yummy salad dressing?

"You're going to have this party next year. Aren't you, Rachel?" Dawn says and grins.

Next year? Next year? How breezily she mentions next year. For half a second the thought of next year sideswipes me and I sway and glance at Rachel and wonder if she detects my thoughts because she walks over and rubs my back and says, "Of course," and smiles that radiant smile and offers us more of everything.

Then Rachel is handing out champagne flutes and we're all huddled around the TV and the ball is dropping and the champagne is popping and we're toasting and kissing and hugging and cheering and giggling—and I'm thinking, Of course, we're all going to be here next year and the year after that and Bush will be out of office . . . and we can toast to that and we'll all grow old together.

It's the week before my one-year checkup and I realize while I've been telling myself I'm okay about it and not obsessing too much and taking it all in stride, I'm making as few plans as possible, only the absolute necessities, nothing frivolous, no dinner plans, no coffees, nothing to make "The Gods" think I'm taking my health and the future for granted. I write everything for the new year on the edges of the December calendar and plan to buy a new calendar after the appointment. If I'm okay.

The days before my one-year checkup, I try to live like a monk—meditate and do yoga and have only calm, blissful thoughts. But life keeps getting in the way.

All week Anna and Maddy fight over who borrowed what and Anna and Alex fight over TV because Alex wants to watch ESPN and Anna is sick of the constant sports banter. Maddy and Alex fight over who touched who at the dinner table, and I wonder why they can't see how silly and petty they are to fight over clothes and TV and personal space when I'm calculating and contemplating my risk of recurrence and how any bad news would impact all of us.

Then I realize it's good. Good that their lives have returned to such a state of normalcy that they can fight over nothing and obviously aren't worrying about me.

The dishwasher leaks and Mike claims it's because I don't know how to load it (which turns out not to be true, it's actually a faulty pump) but that leads to a bigger fight about how I always feel he's disappointed with my housekeeping skills . . . and he claims I'm just not trying hard enough.

"You try picking up the house all day and having it still look like a disaster."

"Just admit it," he says, "you suck at housework."

"I don't aspire to excel at it and if I'd done less housework and more writing, I'd probably have a book contract by now."

"And I could retire," he says with a twinge of sarcasm. And I think maybe he thinks I'm going to be okay this time because he isn't being as nice as before.

All the middle-aged women in the world are reading and talking about Nora Ephron's *I Feel Bad About My Neck* and I want to feel bad about my neck. I do. But my mind races with all sorts of morbid thoughts and I feel bad I may not ever get to feel bad about my neck. I make bargains with God. *If you help me get past this end-of-life crisis so I can have a midlife crisis, I'll always be loving and kind and patient and compassionate and I need to be okay because I can't bear the idea of distracting the kids or Mike any more than I already have.*

The night before my appointment I eat organic brussels sprouts thinking *that* will make a difference, and pretend to meditate because I'm afraid to sleep.

In pitch black we drive to Mayo for my appointment, the light from our headlights carving a narrow path through the dim. I stare out the window and count illuminated mile markers and think, I don't want Mike to lose me, because he hates losing things and I hate being lost so it really wouldn't work out for either of us.

"If I'm okay," I say after I play that thought out in my mind several more times, "I want to go to Italy. I've always wanted to go there."

Mike nods, his face tight as he stares out the windshield and says nothing.

I go back to counting mile markers.

"And if I'm not okay, . . . " I say, "I *still* want to go to Italy."

He says nothing at first and I wonder if he's heard me and then he turns to me and says, "I guess we're going to Italy."

As I sit in the mammogram waiting room in my stiff padded chair, waiting to be either called back or told to go, I think about my right breast, the one that's been biopsied too many times. I figure its days are numbered. But I've grown oddly attached to it this past year. It's my underdog, my handicap, my Achilles' heel, my proof of survival and I realize I'm rooting for it. But I also know, if I have to let it go, I'll get the best damn rack available—Jennifer Aniston's rack—and I'll flaunt it every chance I get.

But I am okay. All clear. No repeat films. No biopsies.

I jump up and hug everyone in the place. My technician, the receptionist, another woman who's just been given the all clear. I feel like I've won the lottery. Only the prize isn't money—it's life. Sort of like the reverse of the Shirley Jackson short story. No public stoning for me today.

In the outer waiting room, I find Mike dozing in a chair and rush up to him and throw my arms around his neck and say, "I'm okay and I'm sorry you had to wake up so early to come here with me and that I've dragged you through all this and that I've been driving you crazy with my fears and that. . . . "

I'm about to say I'm sorry that I don't know how to do this marriage thing right and I don't know if I ever will and I'm sorry if he's disappointed with the way his life turned out with me. . . .

But he stands and hugs me back, his soft cotton shirt soothing against my cheek, and I let him.

"You don't have to apologize," he says, holding me tight against his chest.

"Thanks for saying that," I say.

In the car I'm chattering the entire way about buying a new calendar and our trip to Italy and getting together with friends and taking Dawn a stack of books I promised her on New Year's Eve and that pasta pesto I know she likes and maybe tomorrow I'll waste some time reading a junky magazine and did I ever tell him that one of my best memories of us together was when we went grocery shopping once and I glanced over at him squeezing melons and something about that really turned me on and he laughs and the sun at our backs is unseasonably strong, determined to shine, a golden talisman in the sky, guiding us all the way home.

· · ·

Back in Madison that evening, I kiss the children repeatedly, telling them I'm fine! I'm fine! I'm fine! I can't stop saying it! Or thinking in exclamation points!! Then I tell Anna and Maddy that I'm going to Victoria's Secret to buy a new bra as a gift to my boobs.

"You hate the mall," Anna says.

"I know but I just REALLY want a new bra," I say.

"We'll go with you," Maddy says.

We park the car near the entrance closest to Victoria's Secret, walking past Spencer Gifts and Orange Julius and Auntie Anne's Pretzels and as we take a right at Aveda, I say, "Are you two worried about your own breasts because I'm sorry that I've. . . . "

"It wasn't your fault," Maddy says.

"You have to stop blaming yourself," Anna says.

Their responses don't exactly answer my question and I'm not convinced they aren't worried and I worry that I've altered our relationship irreparably, caused them to mature too fast. Who am I kidding? Things are not "back to normal," probably never will be, but I don't probe any further. Not today.

Once we're inside the store, they leave me in the Just Pink section and head over to the newest bra collections in back. I look for and find the wall of cotton under-wires I always wear and study the choices, thinking maybe I'll buy a white *and* a black, or maybe a tan, when Anna and Maddy surround me.

"Put those bras down," Maddy says, grabbing them out of my hand and pulling me by the elbow over to the Very Sexy collection.

Maddy reaches up for a purple lacy see-through, ut-terly slutty-looking bra and places it in my hand and says, "This is the one."

They both nod.

"I never wear bras like this," I say, shaking my head.

"And that's exactly why you should," Maddy says.

"Exactly," Anna says.

I don't say anything for a second and try to picture myself in it and I wonder how it would make me feel. Would it make me more self-conscious or less? Would it emphasize my imperfections or enhance them? Is this taunting "The Gods" and putting my next checkup at risk? Or is this my way of saying, Screw you cancer, you can't have these puppies . . . not yet and I'm gonna show them off, flaws and all?

The girls are looking at me, waiting for my reply.

Finally I say, "Does it come with matching boy-cut undies, like the ones Carrie wore in *Sex and the City?*"

On the way home I ask the girls, "Would you guys run the NYC Half-Marathon with me in August? I was thinking we should do it together this year."

"I hate racing, " Anna says. "I mean, I race for cross-country and I hate those races and more racing? And thirteen miles? I don't think I can run thirteen miles."

"You know I don't even like running," Maddy says, shaking her head. "That sounds like pure torture to me."

What they say isn't entirely true. But the three of us *do* have a complex and, at times, tortuous relationship with running. It all started years ago when I tried to get Anna to run with me. Whenever I asked her to join me, she'd say, no she would *never* run. It was so BORING. Then a few months after I stopped asking, she said she wanted to start running.

At first it was hard. She couldn't run very far. Maybe five minutes and then we'd walk and she'd complain; her legs hurt, her side hurt, how long has it been, and why was I making her do this? My runs, which had been my escape, were now spent telling her she could do it and it's better not to ask how long and explaining that runners run through the pain.

It was frustrating and not very fun but slowly, gradually we worked up to longer periods of running, with less complaining. By the time Anna could run a few miles without stopping, Maddy said *she* wanted to run and I was back to getting her started.

Then one miraculous day we were all able to run the same distance, the same speed. And running became something we did together on weekends and vacations, a way to spend uninterrupted time. Sweating and panting and breathing in unison lowered all of our defenses and that was when we talked, really talked. When they both went out for cross-country, I was ecstatically happy and proud, considering what a nonathlete I'd been until my late thirties. I secretly felt as if *I'd* made the team. And while every run isn't always ideal (there are times the run is all about them dumping frustration on the trail that usually ends up on me), still I love that we have this to share. Perhaps getting them hooked on running was my finest moment of motherhood . . .

"Oh come on, girls," I say now. "We'll take a few extra days and have fun in New York and we can train together. I mean, Maddy and I can train here and you can train at college," I say to Anna, "but we can all talk about it. It'll be something to share and we'll get in really good shape and the thing is . . . I'd just really like to do it with both of you."

They exchange a look that I know means they don't *really* want to but they know how much it means to me and they both say yes.

twenty-five

Valentine's Day
with
My Shirt On

I T'S A YEAR and two weeks since my surgery and I'm sitting with Mike, Maddy, and Alex at Dotty Dumpling's on Valentine's Day in my purple bra, celebrating our family's ten-year anniversary in Madison. I recall the day we rode into town, a decade ago, with a puppy and a baby and two little girls and our whole lives ahead of us and the first thing I noticed were hearts in all the store windows and I wondered, What's with all the hearts?

And then it struck me that it was Valentine's Day. I'd been so oblivious and overwhelmed by that mid-year move from Vermont, by doing too much and not any of it with much attention and telling myself that after we got through this, I would finally make my life the way I wanted it to be, that I didn't know what day it was. And I think about a year ago this Valentine's Day, two weeks after my surgery, and all the hearts seemed a mockery of what I'd just been through, a frivolous celebration for those who didn't have to worry about how they were going to live their lives in six-month increments.

But this Valentine's Day I am very aware of what day it is, of what a year we've been through, the good, the bad, and the ugly in this past decade, of how fleeting life is and how not paying attention makes it even more so. Mostly I'm just feeling damn grateful that I'm here, with my shirt on, instead of topless at the oncologist's office.

After we order, I turn to Alex and say, "You still want a puppy?"

"Are you serious?" he says, his eyes wide and disbelieving.

I pause. Am I serious? A puppy is a lot of work. And I know I'll end up taking care of it more than anyone and it'll poop all over the house and ruin our new family room couch (that we *did* end up ordering and will arrive next month) and whine to be let out and need to be walked and cuddled and played with. It'll rest its warm head on my feet as I write (just like our dog who died) and it represents an emotional and actual gesture toward the future that I'm finally, after this tumultuous year, ready to embrace.

I nod, and Alex throws his arms around my waist, buries his head near my chest and Mike (who wants the puppy even more than Alex) grabs both my hands. And I think, *This is living, this is everything that matters and there is no place I'd rather be and nothing I'd rather do than be here with my family hugging into me.*

Then Alex accidentally kicks Maddy, but she's pissed and slugs him (not too hard), but now Alex is crying. And Mike is yelling at Maddy, and I'm yelling at Mike for yelling, asking him if he ever read any of the parenting books I recommended over the past eighteen years, and he looks at me as if I'm speaking in tongues.

Maddy says, "I don't know what I'm doing here, anyway. I'm too busy to go out with you guys, considering it's junior year and I'm taking *the* hardest classes at West because you guys expect me to get into a good college."

"Don't call us 'you guys,'" Mike says and I nod in agreement with that. But then he says, "Yes, we *do* want you to get into a good college. Why wouldn't we want the best for you?"

Alex's eyes are still tearful as he says, "I am so sick of hearing about college. I'm in fifth grade and I don't want to worry about this."

"Don't worry about it," I say.

"I may not go to college," he says.

"See what your 'Don't worry about it' does to the kids? Don't worry about it? It's a competitive world out there," Mike says. "And do you have to undermine my authority every chance you get?"

"I'm not trying to undermine you, but I think you pressuring them isn't the way to go about this. I thought we would do it differently this time. Didn't we learn anything?"

He shrugs.

"I wanted this to be a nice celebration," I say.

"Are you putting this in a column?" Maddy asks. "'Cause I don't want you to make me sound bratty or babyish."

"And don't make me out to be the ogre," Mike says.

"Could you say that I'm a really good baseball player?" Alex asks. "And that my favorite song is 'Bye Bye Miss American Pie'?" He starts singing.

"Tell him to stop," Maddy says.

". . . and I knew if I had my chance. . . . "

"Mom, aren't you going to do anything?" Maddy says.

Alex is still singing.

So the truth is, everything and nothing has changed. My kids fight and the getting-into-college pressure looms again; and Mike and I have issues and I still haven't launched myself; and I have a bum breast and unpredictable cells and scars that will never fully heal.

But, I've got another good five months (until I start worrying about my next checkup) and we *have* launched our oldest daughter; and I've sent her two care packages with the chocolate-covered raisins from the other side of town; and I'm writing and I have a new agent who likes my columns; and we're going to Italy and we're getting a puppy; and I'm wearing my new slutty bra and boy-cut undies (which Mike *really* likes); and I'm still yearning and questing, riding my life like a roller coaster, climbing and plunging with exhilaration on the brink of fear, absorbing it all through a new prism—slightly sharper, more nuanced, brimming with possibilities.

Epilogue
Pink Fucking Frosting

And then . . . on a day I'm feeling euphorically alive, a day so glorious, the sky so clear, the sun so bright I have to squint even with my oversized movie star sunglasses on, a day I'm Ginger Rogers sashaying into the grocery store, I run into Dawn Myers. She's yellowed and prune faced and frail and wincing in pain as she inches her way over and tells me that the cancer's back.

I tell her I'm so sorry. Ask her if there's anything I can do for her. She shakes her head. Then I glance into her cart at the dozen miniature, pink frosted cupcakes, and she says, "It's Claire's birthday tomorrow and she loves pink frosting. . . . "

In my car I have a meltdown: for Dawn and her daughter; for all the mothers who've had to abandon daughters and all the daughters who've been abandoned; for pink fucking frosting; for the fact that someone somewhere is losing someone this very second, a collective grief so overwhelming I can't remember how to start my car.

I'm weeping and shivering, right back where I was when cancer barged its cruel-ass self into my life. It isn't fair. It isn't fair. It isn't. . . . I don't want her to be in pain. I don't want her to suffer. I don't want her to die. Ever ever ever ever everevereverever**ever**. . . . I inch my hand into my purse and root and grope and root and grope for what I'm not sure until I manage to place my trembling fingers on the keys, rattle them into the ignition, turn on the power, put down the top, shift into gear, my hair whipping and knotting in the wind as I crank up my tunes, and belt out "Beast of Burden" at the top of my lungs, singing and crying as far as the road will take me.

Postscript

It's June. Two days before we leave for Venice. Haven't seen Dawn in a while. Left phone messages. Dropped off another stack of books. Door always open. Nobody ever home.

Call Rachel (who I know has seen Dawn) and tell her I want to take Dawn out on Mike's motorboat and get her stoned before we leave the country. She laughs but agrees to call Dawn. Call Polly to get the pot. She says she can drop it off but can't go with us. Rachel calls back and says that Dawn would love to go on the boat but no pot. She wants to stay as healthy as possible since there's another procedure she might still be eligible for. At the boat launch, Rachel drives her van to the edge of the dock and we help Dawn out of the car. Her legs are swollen from liver malfunction, her face aged a decade since early spring, her body nearly heftless as we hoist her into the boat. Mike takes off too fast and I worry the wind will topple her and I whisper to Mike, "Slow down. It might be too much. . . . " "No," Dawn says and I turn around to see her face tilted toward the sky, her mouth open wide and smiling. Radiating joy. "Faster," she says. "Faster. Faster."

End of July checkup: My breast MRI is normal but they inadvertently detect a few spots on my liver that they think are cysts.

"Probably nothing to worry about," my doctor says.

But she recommends an ultrasound just to make sure. Mike and I decide it would be easiest to have him do one back in Madison instead of driving all the way back to Mayo, especially since I'm leaving for New York City for the half-marathon in less than a week.

A few days later, Mike and Alex and I go to the hospital (just before heading out to Alex's and my favorite Laotian restaurant for dinner). Alex sits in a chair in the corner of the ultrasound room as I climb on the table and Mike rubs goo on my belly. Just like he used to do when I was pregnant, I'm thinking, remembering how exciting it was to see the heartbeat, to confirm the life growing inside me, when I look up at his face and see his eyes squinting into the screen, his forehead squeezed too tight, his lips sealed into a hard line.

"What? What is that look?" I ask.

He rolls the doppler over my belly, presses in harder, shoves it up under my ribcage.

"Ouch! You're hurting me," I say.

He eases up a tiny bit. Says nothing.

"Why aren't you saying anything?" I say, my voice rising as Alex rises from his chair and walks over to the screen.

"It isn't cysts," Mike says to me.

"So what is it?" I ask.

He presses down harder again and stares at the screen. No reply.

"Tell me!" I say. "Tell me what you're thinking."

Alex is pacing now.

"Get him out of here," I say. "We shouldn't be doing this. Not in front of him."

"Go sit down," Mike says to Alex.

"What?" I mouth to Mike.

"What do you think?" he mouths back.

"Cancer in my liver?" I mouth.

Mike keeps staring at the screen. "Probably hemangiomas but . . . we'll need to schedule an MRI to confirm," he says.

"Hemangioma? What the hell is that?"

"A benign cluster of blood vessels."

"I don't have time for this. I'm going to New York with the girls," I say. "I can still run the race, can't I?" I've been running. I run. I can run. . . .

He turns off the machine, hands me tissues to wipe the goo off my belly and all I can think is, I promised the girls. Promised them. Must keep my promise.

We go to dinner because . . . it's dinnertime, even though nothing seems solid enough to mark. Time an artificial construct devised by people who had too much of it to taunt those who don't.

And this, this is NOT how I want the story to end. Not at all, is what I'm thinking when Alex says, "Aren't you going to eat your squash curry, Mom?" His voice so gentle, so sweet, I feel my throat constrict and worry that I will never swallow again. "That's your favorite," he reminds me. Fakes a grin.

I look down and see that I've been pushing my squash and Japanese eggplant around my plate, thinking about my liver. My liver? I never gave my liver much thought. I'd been thinking it was all about my breasts. What a fool to think I could outthink this.

Mike stares into his plate of food, looking so grim that I'm sure he MUST know something he's not telling me.

"Are you not telling me something?" I hiss under my breath.

He doesn't answer. Goddamned WASPy restraint making me CRAZY.

"What are you not telling me?"

Small talk from other tables and the sound of forks scraping plates my only reply.

"Tell me! Tell me!" I say, too loud. Too emotionally. Too frightened. Too freaked. This is wrong. All wrong. In front of Alex. *This* is my worst mothering moment and I don't know what to do.

But I try to redeem something, try to find the center I feel disintegrating. I lower my voice, turn my head to Mike, and say, "If it *is* bad [I mouth 'bad'], I can't do it like this. I can't have you not answering me. I can't have us assuming the worst and scaring the children [I mouth 'children']."

"I shouldn't have been involved like this," Mike says, shaking his head. "I shouldn't have done the ultrasound."

"But you did and you are and now we have to deal with what is."

"This is about me, too," Mike says, his eyes softening, his lips parting, unsure, and I see how much this has taken him by surprise, how ill equipped we both are to comfort the other, how tenuously we're hanging on.

"Damn it," I say aloud, and then *fuck fuck fuck fuck* to myself. I don't know how to handle this. Could someone tell me how to handle this?

I glance at Alex and see how hard he is fighting back tears pooling in the corners of his eyes. Fuck, I don't want him to work this hard.

"I'm going to be okay," I say to Alex even as my own tears fall. "I promise. You know I've been training for the race. You know I'm strong."

He nods. A little.

"Wanna arm wrestle?" I say.

He shakes his head. Looks down.

"Tell him I'm going to be okay," I say to Mike.

Mike sort of nods.

"Tell him I'm okay!"

Alex's face is redder now and he's gnawing at his lower lip, trembling. How much worse can this get?

I glare at Mike.

"She'll be fine," Mike mumbles mechanically.

I grab both of Alex's hands into mine and ask him, "What's upsetting you, honey? That we're fighting or that you're worried about me?"

"Both," he says and yanks his hands away and presses them against his eyes.

"I am going to be okay," I say. "I promise." And wonder what kind of long-term damage those two words could cause.

A day later I'm back on the ultrasound table with a technician who shares my hairdresser and love of running and confirms the liver spots and that they aren't cysts and also finds some cysts on my kidneys and says I'll need an MRI. What the hell else is going on in there? In between procedures, I overhear Mike suggesting they not use the Gadolinium (the contrast) on me since I had an MRI so recently. He explains that there might be health risks associated with the Gadolinium. More risks. More worries. I'm whisked off to MRI, where I am sucked into a machine that taps avant-garde sounds into my ears. I try to find a pattern in the tapping. I don't. Try to meditate with the mantra I used when I first started yoga. I am. I am. I am. To remind myself I deserve to be. But it turns into No no no no no no. Please no.

And after, I get dressed and wait in the radiology office for Mike. Say hi to Mike's partners who wander in.

I'm not sure what they know or *if* they know but for all of our sakes, I avoid their eyes.

I stare out the window, watch a crane lift and toss cement shards into a dusty heap. Lift and toss and lift and I am so tired from not having slept at all the night before that I'm nearly nodding off when Mike walks in smiling. "We're pretty sure that the spots are benign hemangiomas," he says.

"Really?" I ask.

"As sure as we can be without a CAT scan," he says.

"A CAT scan? You think I need a CAT scan?"

"No, probably not . . . and there's the radiation risk from that. You've had a lot of radiation already. . . . "

"So I'm fine?" I say.

He nods, pretty confidently. "We'll follow you up with an ultrasound in January. But it's probably fine."

"Probably, huh?" I say, wanting more, but trying to find enough in "probably," enough to gather up my things, take Mike's hand, walk out the hospital door, into the parking lot, climb in the car, and get on with my life.

As soon as Alex comes home from school, I scoop him up in my arms even though I can barely lift him, his heft surprising and delighting me, and I say, "I'm okay. I'm fine. I'm healthy. I'm sorry."

He smiles his heartbreaking, broad, gap-toothed smile, his face full of hope and faith and belief in me, and he buries his head in my neck and snuggles in just like he did when he was a baby and wanted to be held all day, and I am so grateful that I can *say* these words, that I *didn't* break my promise, that our embrace obscures how desperately *I* need to believe.

Dawn Myers died peacefully in her home filled with family and friends on August 5, 2007. Seven hours earlier, my daughters and I crossed the New York City Half-Marathon finish line.

Acknowledgments

My heartfelt gratitude to everyone who encouraged me to write. Ever.

To Kristy Kiernan and Lolly Winston, who both said I had to do something with the crazy CANCER IS A BITCH essay I sent them on an impulsive whim. To Majorie Osterhout and *Literary Mama* for taking a chance on me and offering me a column based on that essay. To the readers I found at *Literary Mama,* who responded so generously and soulfully to my words. All of you gave me the courage to share my story openly and intimately.

To Larry Weissman and Sascha Alper, who believed me when I said I could write a book and magically coaxed me to discover its essence. You are agents and confidants of the highest order; brilliant, honorable, and worldly-wise.

To my wonderful editor at Da Capo Press, Wendy Francis. Your edits rocked! To Christine Arden, copyeditor extraordinaire! And Renee Caputo, for your patience with me.

To my manuscript readers and writing buddies, in addition to Kristy, Lolly, Larry, and Sascha, I thank

Alexandria Brown Baker, Richard Joint Baker Jr., Caroline Grant, Caitlin Jane Berry, Rachel Sarah, and the rest of the *Literary Mama* columnists, as well as Bridget Birdsall, Autumn Arnold, Miki Knezevic and the SAMIs, Mark Wisniewski, Amy MacKinnon, Eileen Cook, Danielle Younge-Ullman, Jenny Gardiner, Jess Riley and Lisa Daily, Peggy Towers, Jim Robertson, the two Janes (and all my other Sewanee friends). Thank you all for your honest feedback and unwavering support.

To my friends, a list that is deep and sustaining. In addition to all of the above, Marie Heiligenstein and Roseanne Clark (my soul sisters), Yael Gen, Katie Middleton, Peggy Scanlon, Mark Frankel, Gina Golding, Carla Raushenbush, all my running and yoga buddies and my friends and neighbors who brought me flowers and meals and homemade cookies and helped me out with my kids after my surgery. Your loving kindness floored me, helped me *and* my family heal. Thank all of you for laughing and crying and sharing life with me.

To my family. . . . Just writing the word "family" chokes me up. Thank you Rick and Ali and Abby and Andrew for existing (that alone seems a miracle to me). Thank you for filling our home with your unique and spirited auras, for accepting mine, for understanding all the times I didn't make dinner, couldn't find the soccer socks, or pads, *or* cleats. For all the times I had my head buried in my computer, chose writing over relaxing with you. Thank you Rick, for more than two decades of love and loyalty and passionate exchange, for stopping me every time I thought I should quit, for understanding my need to write this story, for accepting the all of me. Each one of you has sacrificed so I could realize my dream. I've learned that's the way it is when you live with and love people, when you have a family and I stand in awe, beyond grateful.

Thank you is not enough.

·